THE HEALING

POWER

OF

ESSENTIAL OILS

THE ORIGINAL LIQUID COPALS

BEVONNE BIRCH CROOKSTON

In order that all may know this signifies that,

Bevonne Birch Crookston, Paway – yatanatu way - akt,

Is a member in good standing of the Oklevueha Band and Native American Traditional Organization as a Native American Practitioner and Traditional Spiritual Leader of the Band.

Her current designation is:

Medicine Woman

As such, she is empowered to perform her duty as a Healer to the best of her knowledge and understanding and, so long as she continues to uphold the conditions of her covenant, she is upheld in her calling by the Elders and Councils of the Oklevueha Band and Native American Traditional Organization.

In order to remove all doubt, I do attest to the same this 3rd day of July, 2009.

Man Found Standing – Principle Medicine Chief

Paul H. Dean – Oklevueha Band

FOREWORD

In 2004 the United States government passed a law regulating how the citizens of the United States can talk about the healing properties of plants. In the USA the essential oils are considered an over-the-counter drug and the average person cannot use the term "essential oils" when describing the healing properties of plants. The Native Americans, however, still have that right. In 2003 I was adopted as a Medicine Woman into the Nemenhah Band and in 2009 into the Oklevueha Band. As a Medicine Woman, I am able to share my knowledge of the benefits of our sacred healing plants. In this book, I will refer to the liquid plant extracts as both essential oils, as other countries around the world call them, or as liquid copals using the Native American term.

Many years ago a friend gave me a book about the benefits of herbs that sparked my interest. I was excited to know God had given us healing plants and I wanted to know everything I could about them. I couldn't put the book down. It was like I had finally come upon the path my spirit wanted to follow. When I told my mother how this new knowledge made me feel, she told me about my great-grandmother's ability to use the traditional healing plants to benefit her family and community. I felt so connected with my grandmother and longed for her knowledge.

I began reading and taking notes from every available book on the healing properties of plants. I attended workshops, listened to cassette tapes, watched videos, and started using the herbs. In 1992 I was introduced to the essential oils. This was exciting for me as I saw the traditional healing taken to another level.

In 1993 my husband, Rex, and I were able to volunteer and spend three months on an herb farm in Idaho. We helped with the planting and weeding of the Lavender, Clary Sage, Peppermint, and Thyme. We loved seeing the plants in bloom and smelling the fragrance as we worked in the fields.

We learned that it is not easy to grow organic crops. During the next few years, I met people who were just getting started using the essential oils and they requested a copy of my notes. Thanks to my daughter, Lark, and my sister, Vallejo, we printed the first edition of "Bevonne's Notebook" in 1996. In 2006 I added additional workbooks, DVDs, and CDs to assist others in learning and applying the oils.

I would like to thank all those who have touched my life and all those from whom I have gathered knowledge. This Workbook is a reflection of the influence of others. Every day I find ways the oils bless my life. Sometimes it is little things like taking care of mosquito bites and other times it has been quite major, like saving my husband's life from carbon monoxide poisoning in 1995. In 2003 Rex passed away from Malaria complications he developed while in Africa.

In September of 2012 I married David Crookston and together we are continuing teaching about the healing powers of the essential oils. It is nice to again have someone working with me. I hope this Workbook will help you learn about the sacred liquid copals and their traditional uses. May you learn to love them as much as I do.

Bevonne Birch Crookston - Medicine Woman
Bevonne25@Yahoo.com

IMPORTANT! The information contained in this workbook is intended for educational purposes only and was gathered for the personal use of the compiler. The essential oils referenced to herein are pure sacred liquid copals. The material in this document was obtained from lectures, tapes, videos, books, and my personal experiences. It is not provided in order to diagnose, prescribe or treat any disease, illness or injured condition of the body. Furthermore, the compiler of neither this document, nor any maker or distributor of liquid copals, assumes responsibility for such use. Anyone suffering from any disease, illness or injury should consult with a physician or health care provider.

WORDS TO PONDER

One night I dreamed I was teaching a workshop and I was quoting the words from a song by Will L. Thompson. These are the words:

Have I done any good in the world today? Have I helped anyone in need? Have I cheered up the sad, or made someone feel glad? If not, I have failed indeed.

Has anyone's burdens been lightened today, because I was willing to share? Have the sick and the weary been helped on their way? When they needed my help was I there?

Then wake up and do something more than dream of your mansions above. Doing good is a pleasure, a joy beyond measure, a blessing of duty and love.

There are chances for work all around just now, opportunities right in our way. Do not let them pass by, saying, "sometime I'll try," but go and do something today.

'Tis noble of man to work and to give, love's labors have merit alone. Only he who does something helps others to live. To God each good work will be known.

Then wake up and do something more than dream of your mansions above. Doing good is a pleasure, a joy beyond measure, a blessing of duty and love.

I woke up and pondered the questions. Have I done any good in the world today? Have I cheered up the sad? I have decided to ask myself these questions often and make them a part of my life. Each day I want to do something to lift and build another.

It was Ben Franklin who said that an investment in knowledge pays the best interest. The difference between Franklin's time and ours is that it's becoming increasingly difficult to make a living without continuous learning. This is because we live and work in a global, information-based economy where knowledge is king.

Those who move ahead are the ones who take what they learn and turn it into marketable products, services, and information. Your chances of moving ahead depend heavily on your commitment to lifelong learning. You don't need an advanced degree or professional credentials unless your choice of business requires them, but you do need to master the art of applied learning and make it an integral part of your life.

There's an abundance of information to be had on almost any business you would like to learn, but remember, simply learning what to do is of little value and meaningless until you put it into action.

An anonymous entrepreneur once wrote, "To look is one thing. To see what you look at is another. To understand what you see is a third. To learn from what you understand is still something else, but to act on what you learn is all that really matters." Good ideas are only given to you for a limited amount of time. If you don't act on them, they belong to someone else.

See everything you do in life, including your business, as play. If it isn't play at some level, you are not happy and are squelching your creativity. One way to keep your creativity growing is by doing something each month to push you out of your comfort zone. Is there something you have always wanted to do but are afraid of trying? I challenge you to put on the Confidence liquid copal, stretch yourself, and go to work. I would be interested in hearing about your experience. – Bevonne

CONTENTS

INTRODUCTION TO ESSENTIAL OILS

Natural plant medicines have been used throughout history. They deserve serious study, for their potential as a healing therapy is enormous. Unfortunately, the public today is still largely unfamiliar with how to use plant medicines. The Native Americans have been using plant copal medicines for thousands of years. Natural plant copals are safe, comparatively inexpensive, practical to use, quick acting and effective. Their use to combat infections is adequately documented in medical and scientific literature. There is now sufficient clinical experience to show how plants can be effective for a wide range of health problems. Unfortunately, much of the relevant research and medical literature on this topic is available only in other countries.

As you probably have already come to understand, the alternative health industry is rampant with hype and inferior products. The world's experts are actively engaged in the sham of essential oils testing, certifications, adulteration and misinformation. It can be a daunting task to locate high quality and truly pure therapeutic oils.

The information in this chapter will give you a better understanding about how to choose a supplier and understand the quality differences in the essential oils marketplace.

In France, for instance, many medical doctors use essential oils and herbs to fight common infections. The most common uses are for infections of the respiratory and digestive systems, the urinary tract, the reproductive organs and the skin. The French are world leaders in the use of essential oils for therapeutic purposes and, because it is considered normal, essential oils are covered by health insurance plans. French pharmacies also carry formulas consisting of essential oils and herbal tinctures that are specifically made under a doctor's prescription. Aromatherapy, a name coined by a French chemist, is taught in their colleges,

universities and medical schools. In the United States, although natural plant medicines are commonly available, medical doctors rarely use them in treatments.

The American public, in general, is unfamiliar with essential oils and the possibility of using them for medical purposes. There is comparatively little public or private funding available for natural health care research. In order to make better decisions, people should be informed about alternative treatments and what they can do to live a longer and healthier life. A freely informed public is in everyone's best interest.

As early as 1534, Indians living in Canada showed the French how to counteract scurvy by boiling a mixture of pine needles and white pine bark, a plant rich in Vitamin C. Because of their fixed beliefs, the French did not take the advice and European sailors continued to die from scurvy until well into the nineteenth century. Could our fixed beliefs possibly be getting in the way of progressing to better health?

Essential oils are the end result of plant metabolism, the biological activity of plants. They are synthesized by the plant's chemistry and circulate through the stems, leaves, flowers and roots. They contain the elements that make each plant unique – the scent and the intelligence of the plant. Walk through a forest of pine trees and you can easily smell their fragrance. Essential oils are found in the skin of an orange, in the leaves of a peppermint plant, and in the petals of a rose flower. The plant's aroma and flavor come from their essential oils.

Essential oils are "essential" for a plant's survival. Oils are a key component of the immune system of plants. Scientists have observed that plants use their essential oils for various reasons such as repelling unwanted insects, healing when the plant is injured, preventing water loss from foliage when the climate is hot or dry, and attracting bees and other insects that assist with pollination.

Essential oils are stored by plants in oil and resin ducts, hollow spaces, and cells. They can be found in various parts of the plant such as the leaves, stems, bark, needles, resin, flowers, fruits, and roots. With few exceptions, essential oils are extracted from plant materials through steam distillation or cold pressing. When the oil is distilled, each plant has unique requirements in terms of how it should be handled. These include when to harvest, the time between harvesting and distillation, distillation equipment, temperature, pressure, and when to stop distillation in order to avoid exposing the extracted oil to excessive heat, thus destroying vital constituents or medicinal properties. The cold pressing is used to remove the citrus oils from the peel of citrus fruits such as grapefruit, orange, lemon, and tangerine.

Thousands of tons of essential oils are used each year by the flavor and fragrance industries. They are inferior in quality to the essential oils used for therapeutic purposes. Because of the limited amount of plants grown in the world each year, many commercial growers will use various methods to make growing more profitable for them. They will use chemicals for growing the plants and extreme heat, pressure, or chemical solvents to squeeze more liquid from the plants during distillation. These processes not only cut production time and reduce costs, but they also greatly compromise the quality being produced.

These practices result in oils with very little (if any) life force left in them. Many times, the very small trace constituents that are lost are the ones most important for healing. The oil may still have a flavor or fragrance to satisfy the perfume and food industry, but they are not the quality essential oils necessary for healing. In fact, this lower standard is very acceptable for flavoring or fragrance. Since the demand for therapeutic grade essential oils comprises less than 5% of the market, it is the suppliers that buy the food and perfume grade

essential oils and sell them as "therapeutic" grade who are committing fraud.

Because healing oils are expensive to produce, fraud is rampant in the essential oil industry. At the present time there are no well-regulated labeling laws in the U.S. Because of this, essential oils that say "100%" can mean as little as 10% of the pure oil with the rest being a colorless, odorless chemical. This is considered acceptable in the retail trade.

"Organic" is another misleading term. To an organic chemist any "carbon compound" is considered organic since his definition of organic means, "composed of carbon compounds." So to an organic chemist, gasoline, rubbing alcohol, and dioxin (known to cause cancer) are considered "organic." When these adulterants are added to an essential oil, the term "organic" can still be legally used. That is why it is important to understand who is using the term and be aware of what their definition means. To an unsuspecting customer, many of these odorless, colorless, cheap petrochemicals may be very harmful to their health when applied to the skin or inhaled over a period of time.

It is important to understand the term "aromatherapy grade" originated in England and is known to be the practice of massage with essential oils. To the English, "aromatherapy grade" oil consists of only 2 - 5 % pure essential oil (which can be food or fragrance grade and still meet the English requirement) and 95 - 98% carrier oil. But in America many take the term "aromatherapy grade" to mean pure or therapeutic quality essential oil, which may not be the case. Here is an area where you will need to determine which English is being spoken-- American English or British English. You will soon recognize that when essential oils are labeled "aromatherapy grade" it is probably by definition adulterated and/or diluted.

Most users of essential oils in Britain are horrified at the thought of applying pure, "neat" oils to the body for fear of a toxic reaction. This may be because most British essential oils are by-products of the food and fragrance industry and such oils probably are toxic if used neat. Because only 2 – 5% is used in the "aromatherapy grade," no serious reactions are usually noted. Also, the British do not report the healings that are common in the U.S. and France, both of which are countries where neat therapeutic grade oils are used.

The term "Pure USP Grade Oil" refers to a set of standards for essential oils set by the fragrance and food industries. These standards were set so that all batches of oils will be as identical as possible for use in receipts and formulations. The "USP Grade Oil" is intended for the fragrance and food industry and not for healing.

Another term that can be misleading is "natural." Any compound found in nature that can be produced synthetically by a laboratory can legally be labeled and sold as "natural," even when it is completely unnatural according to my definition. Even though the natural and synthetic compounds would be identical for a specific compound, nature has a way of arranging its chemical properties at a molecular level that can not be duplicated. God makes therapeutic essential oils. All we can do is extract it as lovingly as possible and find a producer who is willing to leave them untouched. God's gift of oils can never be copyrighted, trademarked, or patented for profit. Every person has the right to experience true essential oils.

Throughout the world a pure synthetic methylsalecylate is labeled and sold as natural Wintergreen or Birch Bark. The synthetic will never be able to duplicate the healing properties of the pure essential oil of Wintergreen or Birch Bark. Man can never reproduce the quality nature has made, but because of the money that can be made, many laboratories and skillful chemists are imitating the chemical composition of natural oils. Many of these laboratories are found in France where there is a reputation for excellent oils. There are some French businessmen who produce cheap imitations, label

them "Made in France" and export them knowing they would never meet the high French standards. Some counterfeit oils are so skillfully compounded they are virtually impossible to detect even with the most sophisticated equipment.

Testing laboratories cannot test for every single component because nature contains hundreds of components, most in trace amounts, that have not yet been determined. Skillful chemists know the labs will only test for the 10 or 15 most abundant ingredients contained in natural oils so these are the ones they combine to produce their counterfeit.

When a true, pure oil, and false synthetic oil are tested for their most abundant constituents, they look identical as far as the analysis goes. The synthetic oil is dead and has very little if any healing capability. Only God can give it the life and healing abilities. While the lab cannot tell the difference, if you are not receiving the known benefits mentioned for the pure therapeutic essential oils, you probably do not have the right essential oils.

Dr. Herve Casabianca, director of the largest essential oil testing laboratory in France, has come to the conclusion that it is important to "know your grower, know your distiller, and know your supplier." He says, "The chemists have become so clever that they can sometimes fool even the best testing laboratories."

While commercial essential oils in the flavor and fragrance industry are routinely adjusted, blended, redistilled, or adulterated, essential oils used for medicinal purposes should always be a single-species and unaltered from their natural state. That means the liquid in the bottle contains only the distillation of a single plant species, is free from all man-made chemicals including contaminants such as herbicides, and pesticides. The trade of essential oils is worldwide. The same species of a plant grown in different countries under different soil and altitude conditions will produce crops that differ in their chemical makeup and therapeutic properties.

For instance, the Ravintsara grown in Madagascar is far superior to that grown in China. Yet some suppliers will actually mix a little of the quality essential oil with the cheaper oil and sell it for the higher price. It is important to have a supplier that has integrity. When the oil's country of origin is listed on the label, it is another indication it probably hasn't been diluted by the supplier.

There are some 30 different species of Lavender and each has different chemical constituents and medicinal characteristics. On the open market, their quality and price can vary greatly, and certain ones are only used in the flavor and fragrance industry. If the different plant species of Lavender are mixed together and sold under the generic name "Lavender," it becomes difficult to know with certainty what medicinal effect, if any, this mixture will have. In contrast, the therapeutic qualities of a single species such as *Lavandula vera* are predictable because the characteristics are fully documented and well understood.

When purchasing therapeutic essential oils, insist on the species that produces the best results. There may be a difference in price between Lavender (*Lavandula angustifolia)* and Lavandin (*L. hybrida*), but this difference is meaningless if the less costly essential oil has fewer therapeutic properties. Essential oils are the high-grade fuel of plants and by applying them to our body we receive the best the plants have to offer. They are so flexible and wonderful to use, it is easy to incorporate them into every lifestyle.

Essential oils should always be purchased in protective dark glass bottles (blue bottles being the better choice) with airtight seals. Some scientists believe dark glass bottles protect the oils from light that will destroy the oil's capability to penetrate the skin and bring about healing. The airtight seal prevents oxidation and keeps the volatile components of the oil in the bottle; thereby, retaining their therapeutic properties.

Therapeutic grade oils are not usually sold in retail stores. It is believed over 90% of the "essential oils" sold in the U.S. are fragrance or food grade and unsuitable for healing. I have noticed some books written on essential oils are written by those with little or no experience with therapeutic quality oils. They do not realize the toxicity they may have experienced or read about came from adulterated or synthetic oils. There is so much adulteration in the essential oil industry I want to set the therapeutic grade essential oils apart from the food and fragrance grade essential oils. The essential oils are very powerful and must be used with respect, in small amounts, and are best diluted with carrier oil when you first begin using them.

There are oils which, when mixed together, mimic the aroma of a more expensive oil. For example, Carnation oil is very expensive, so Black Pepper and Ylang Ylang are combined to create the aroma of carnation. Unscrupulous suppliers will dilute a pure essential oil in a carrier base and pass it off as pure natural essence. Those essential oils combined with carrier oil are the easier to spot than other dilutions because the base oil is oily. Neat essential oils for the most part are not oily. Again, it is good to know your supplier and the source of their essential oils.

Diffusing the oils is another way to enjoy the full benefits of their aromatic influences. I use them "neat" (pure/undiluted) in a diffuser to either purify the air or set a specific mood in the home. I will use Purify, Spice Traders, or Joyful when there is sickness in the family. These oils keep the airborne bacteria and viruses in check. When my home is filled with grandchildren, I diffuse Citrus Plus or Serenity to keep the mood happy and calm. These oils also work well to calm a stressful day. When I am studying or doing taxes I like to diffuse Lemon or Focus. If I want a more romantic mood there are several oils to choose from such as Balance, Love, or Passion for Life.

Diffusing the essential oils not only removes dust

particles out of the air but is also a great air filtration system. Until I purchased a diffuser, I used 15 drops of oil in a two ounce spray bottle filled with water, shook and sprayed around the room. This is also a good way to use the oils when traveling to purify the hotel room, keep the driver alert, or calm the children. As you use the oils, you will wonder how you ever tolerated the chemical substitutes.

For quick applications I will use the oils on the bottom of my feet, on my wrists, and ears. I really enjoy using about six drops of the oils in a warm bath. For my face I use various oils such as Rose Blend, Cucumber, Frankincense, Myrrh, Rosemary, Sandalwoods, Baby Soft (I always dilute in carrier oil because it is hot on my skin), Freedom, and Skin Care. As you read through the various essential oils, note which ones may be beneficial for your skin type.

There are specific Vita Flex points related to certain areas of the body on the feet (see Vita Flex Chart). Sometimes I apply the oils on specific areas of the feet as well as on the Energy Centers (or Chakras). The main energy centers are located on the top of the head, center of forehead, throat area, center of chest, above the naval, lower abdomen, and base of the spine (coccyx). There are also powerful energy centers in the palm of each hand and on the sole of each foot. You will find more information on the Energy Centers under the Nutritional Tips & Information Section of this book.

HERE ARE SOME GUIDELINES FOR USING ESSENTIAL OILS:

- Educate yourself about essential oils. Keep oils, absolutes, synergies, and blends out of reach of children.

- Do not, unless otherwise advised by an expert, apply neat essential oils onto the skin.

- Never assume that oils will have the same properties as credited to the whole plant from which it is obtained. Some oils can be up to 100,000 times stronger than the dried herb.

- Essential oils should always be used diluted over a large body area.

- Regulate the frequency when using essential oils. If used daily over a two-week period, give a week's grace before recommencing treatment.

- Reduce the chance of acquiring a sensitivity reaction from constant use of the same oil over several years by varying choices. This gives the body a break from constant use.

- If any kind of skin rash is observed when using a particular essential oil, stop use immediately, and wait a few days before trying another oil.

- Some oils may be **hot** when applied to the skin. Hot oils to use with **caution** are Birch Bark, Cinnamon Bark, Wintergreen, Clove Buds, Eucalyptus globulus, Oregano, Thyme, and Peppermint. Remember everyone is different. What is not hot to one person may be very hot for another. I've noticed that when a person's pH is acidic then oils seem to be hotter for them.

- If an essential oil feels **hot** when applied to the skin, use carrier oil to dilute it. Keep applying more carrier oil until the burning stops. It is good to always have a small bottle of carrier oil in your kit to use if the oil is hot when applied. **Never use water to dilute a hot essential oil because it will only make the oil hotter on the skin.** Essential oils do not dissolve in water. They must be diluted with some type of vegetable or carrier oil.

- When diluting essential oils in carrier oil (cold pressed vegetable oil) the general rule is to use six drops of the pure oil to ¼ ounces of carrier oil. Generally, using more than six to eight drops of the pure essential oil is wasting it.

- Never use mineral oil or baby oil as a massage base. They are toxic to the body. Mineral oil is a petro-chemical, refined from gasoline, very hard on the skin, and the essential oil may fight against it. It also will rob your vitamin supply.

- **Essential Oils must be kept out of the eyes!** If they get into the eyes **do not** use water to wash them out. Use a pure vegetable oil. Do not handle contact lenses or rub eyes with the essential oils on your fingers. Oils with high phenol content like Oregano, Cinnamon Bark, Clove Buds, Thyme, Lemongrass, or Bergamot may damage contacts and irritates eyes.

- If you want to use a little essential oil in the ears put it on a cotton swab to apply. **Do not drop oils directly into the ears under any circumstance!!**

- When using the essential oils for the first time, it is best to use only two or three diluted oils until you see how your body is going to respond. Too many oils may encourage the cells to detoxify causing diarrhea.

- Essential oils do not need to be taken internally for good results. In one test a Japanese researcher found that smelling the essential oils was more effective than digesting them. If you do like to use some oils internally, always dilute them with an oil-soluble liquid like honey or olive oil. I like to use the essential oils in cooking. It's important to remember one drop goes a long way. I find it best to mix 15 drops in ¼ ounce of olive oil and then add a few drops to taste.

- Essential oils maintain their shelf life much longer if kept in dark glass bottles that keep the UV rays out, are kept out of direct sunlight, and away form heat above 90 degrees. Keep the caps tightly closed when not in use. It is also advisable to keep the essential oils off electrical appliances since this may change the frequency of the oil.

- Some essential oils contain constituents that may be photo toxic causing a rash or darker pigmentation when exposed to sunlight or UV rays for up to 3 to 4 days after using. These oils are Angelica, Bergamot, Grapefruit, Lemon, Lime, Tangerine, Mandarin, and Orange.

- It is interesting to note that people often suffer from "civilization illnesses" because they are so used to synthetic aromas that they find the purity and potency of genuine essential oils not particularly attractive. It is best to introduce them to oils with a gentle massage choosing oils whose fragrances are widely accepted such as Lavender or Mandarin. Other oils that harmonize with a basic blend of Mandarin or Lavender are Spikenard, Roman Chamomile, or Clary Sage.

- Pregnant women, epileptics, and those with high blood pressure should consult a health care professional when starting any type of health program.

- People with allergies should test a small amount of oil on a small area of sensitive skin, such as the inside of the arm, before applying the oil on other areas. The bottom of the feet is one of the safest, most effective places to use oils.

- It is best not to add undiluted essential oils directly to bath water. To disperse the oil more evenly add a few drops to a dispersing agent (a bath gel) then add to the bath water.

- Keep neat essential oils away from open flames, sparks, or electricity. Some oils such as Fir, Pine, Orange, and Peppermint are potentially flammable.

- **CAUTION:** Some essential oils can be fatal if taken internally. It has been reported that as little as 5 ml of Eucalyptus globulus can be fatal for infants.

~~~~~~~~~

HOW TO USE THIS BOOK

This book was written for the intent to educate those wishing to learn and use essential oils. For a quick way to look up various problems and find the oils that have been known to assist them, use the Alphabetical Listing and Systems Guide Sections. The oils in these sections are not listed in any specific order. I recommend you refer to the Single Oils and Synergies and Blends sections to find more specific information about each of the oil. This will assist you in choosing the most beneficial oil for you.

Since some people may be allergic to certain oils you will find some that are quite similar in the benefits they provide. This is to provide more people the opportunity to use and enjoy the oils.

As you use the essential oils you will find new applications to add to the list. You may also find you didn't notice the specific benefit mentioned for a certain oil. Essential oils seem to respond individually. Make this your notebook and write in it what has worked for you.

I have had people explain that a certain oils hadn't worked for them. One lady told me she had put Lavender on a burn and the next day she had a rash around the area on her hand. When I questioned her I found she was out of the therapeutic grade of Lavender and had gone to the local store to purchase what they had.

Most essential oils available at the local drug store or health food store will be food and fragrance grade or adulterated and not the quality needed. In almost all cases you will not receive the benefits I explain in this book. If you want the essential oils to work you will need the pure unadulterated ones.

In the book, Advanced Aromatherapy, Kurt Schnaubelt said, "Aromatherapy would not be so attractive if the only thing it offered was a number of quick, simple, and economical solutions. Anyone who uses essential oils once will continue to explore them and will discover the diverse aspects of natural, aromatic essences—relaxation, stress reduction, immune strengthening, preventive cures, personal hygiene, and other steps on the way to healing and staying healthy. Perhaps aromatherapy's greatest asset lies in its ability to demonstrate the link between physical and emotional health to the user."

Using the metaphor of "lighting a candle" this book is from my heart, a sharing of wisdom and insights I have witnessed over the years. Buddha once said, "Thousands of candles can be lit from a single candle, and the life of the candle cannot be shortened. Happiness never decreases by being shared."

Like the candle, I hope this book reaches and lights up the lives of many people wanting to learn about the healing properties of the Essential Oils.

The ideas expressed in this book have been gathered from many sources and are intended for educational purposes only. Have respect for the essential oils; they are very powerful and always remember a little goes a long ways.

ESSENTIAL OILS SINGLES – The Original Pure Liquid Copals

Three main classes of compounds found in the essential oils are Phenylpropanoids (Fee-nal-Pro-pa-noids), Sesquiterpenes (Ses-qio-Ter-pens), and Monoterpenes (Mah-no-Ter-pens). They are unique to the oils because they not only occur naturally in the plants, but they have the intelligence, and capability to benefit our bodies. Essential oils are powerful in addressing injuries, illnesses, and disease conditions.

There are hundreds of Phenylpropanoids (also called hemiterpenes) and dozens of varieties of them. They are antiseptic and cleanse the receptor sites of our cells allowing the proper transfer of hormones, peptides, steroids, and other intracellular messengers. This allows the cells to communicate and improve body functions. Sickness results when the cells do not communicate with each other and malfunction. Some essential oils that contain Phenylpropanoids are Clove Bud, Basil, Cinnamon Bark, Oregano, Anise, and Peppermint.

The Sesquiterpenes deliver oxygen molecules to the cells much like hemoglobin does in the blood. With more than 10,000 varieties of Sesquiterpenes, they assist in elevating our moods and spirituality. They can also erase or reprogram miswritten codes in the DNA. Their oxygenating capabilities make them strong supporters of the immune system. Essential oils containing Sesquiterpenes are Cedarwood, Vetiver, Sandalwood, Patchouli, Myrrh, Ginger, Blue Tansy, Cypress, and Frankincense.

The Monoterpenes, with more than 2000 varieties, offer many healing properties. Their most important ability is reprogramming miswritten information in the cellular memory. With improper coding in the DNA cells malfunction and disease results. The essential oils of Galbanum, Angelica Root, Peppermint, Pine, Hyssop, Juniper, Frankincense, Oregano, Spruce, Cypress, and Myrtle contain Monoterpenes.

Essential oils need not be taken internally for good results. Applying the oils topically to the skin or smelling them is usually the best way to use them. Before using oils for the first time, a skin test is recommended since every person's skin sensitivity is different. Apply a drop of the oil to a small area of your forearm and wait a few minutes to see if there is any reaction. If the skin becomes irritated or hot apply carrier oil to the area to dilute it. Carrier oil is any plant oil that is expeller pressed such as extra virgin olive oil, sesame seed oil, or coconut oil. If you do not have carrier oil then apply butter to the hot area. Most people have no problems with the majority of the oils except the hot ones such as Oregano, Cinnamon Bark, Thyme, Clove Bud, Birch Bark, Wintergreen, Peppermint, and Lemongrass.

Use caution when applying the oils on skin that has been exposed to cosmetics, soaps, and cleansers containing synthetic chemicals, especially petroleum-based chemicals. Essential oils may react by wanting to pull these chemicals from the body causing skin irritation, nausea, headaches, or other uncomfortable effects. If this happens, drink water to assist the oils in removing the toxins from your body.

As you begin using the oils, it is best to start with two or three diluted in carrier oil. Use the essential oils in moderation until you know how your body is going to respond. If you experience an adverse reaction to the oils, it is wise to discontinue their use and start an internal cleansing program before resuming regular use. If you have too many toxins it is better to cleanse the colon first so you'll have a place to dump the toxins being removed from the body.

When using the essential oils for food flavoring, it is important to remember they are very concentrated and one or two drops can be equivalent to a full bottle of dried herbs.

The GRAS initials by the oils means the FDA generally regards them as safe to be taken internally as dietary supplements. Some believe the oils of Valerian, Lemon, Grapefruit, Orange, and Tangerine are considered to be more effective when taken orally. I personally feel that unless you are using them specifically for digestion, rubbing directly on the skin is very beneficial. When taking the oils internally, **always** use the best therapeutic quality.

Many of the same species of plants are grown in different parts of the world. It has been found that some oils grown in certain countries have higher properties than the same oil in another location. For instance, Oregano grown wild in Turkey is twice the quality and potency as the commonly used European Oregano. Quality Ravintsara comes from Madagascar. For this reason I have included the country of origin for each of the essential oils.

It is also important to know how the plant is grown, whether it is organic, wild crafted, or organically grown. Many essential oil crops are commercially grown and are usually not the quality you are looking for. These crops are generally used in food and fragrance grade essential oils.

At the end of each single essential oil listed you will see which Synergy or Blend that oil is found in.
~~~~~~~~~

AJOWAN SEED, Organically Grown: India
(Trachyspermum ammi) - Known as Indian Thyme. It is an antiseptic and beneficial for infections, bacteria, viruses, fungus, parasites and nausea used as a tonic. In India it is used as a sedative for whooping cough and toothaches. It assists bronchitis, skin disease, gas, diarrhea, digestive weakness, and cholera. It is a circulatory stimulant. Constituent: Phenols-Monoterpenes. Descriptor: Stimulating, antibiotic, antiseptic, stimulates liver.

ANGELICA ROOT, Organically Grown: India
(Angelica archangelica) – It has been praised for its virtues since antiquity. It assists in improving the immune system and strengthening the heart by stimulating circulation. Some of the things it has been used for in Europe are bronchial ailments, a general lung tonic, to stimulate the lymphatic system (especially to detoxify after an illness), gas, indigestion, and to stimulate the appetite. It is beneficial for contagious diseases such as typhus, yellow fever, malaria, diphtheria, cholera, and is used as a urinary antiseptic. Angelica Root is beneficial for cystitis, is a tonic for the liver and spleen. It controls uric acid, improves pepsin and hydrochloric acid production, is an antispasmodic, diuretic, expectorant, and may have bactericidal and fungicidal properties.

It improves dull and congested skin, psoriasis, and anemia. Angelica Root assists in restoring a sense of smell, overcoming fatigue, migraines, nervous tension and stress-related disorders. It assists in releasing or letting go of negative feelings and brings the memory back to the point of origin before trauma or anger was experienced. It promotes balance, gives us strength to overcome difficulties, and causes distaste for alcohol. Descriptor: Tonic, stimulates liver, aid digestion, decongestant, calming, anticoagulant. Constituent: Monoterpenes Courmarins. Found in Guardian and Balance.

ANISE SEED, Organically Grown: Turkey
(Pimpinella anisum) – GRAS - It has been widely used as a domestic spice. Also assists with colic, indigestion, cramps, flatulence, vomiting, diarrhea, bile secretion, muscle aches, spasms, rheumatism, pulmonary congestion, flu, colds, bronchitis, asthma, frigidity and impotence. It has estrogen-like properties and may induce menstruation, ease painful periods, assists with menopause problems, stimulate milk flow, and assists delivery. Avoid in pregnancy. Descriptor: Antibiotic, antiseptic, anti-spasmodic, sedative. Constituent: Phenols/Ketones. Found in Rejuvenate and Tummy Rub.

ARTEMESIA, Organically Grown: India *(Artemesia annua)* – It is also known as Sweet Annie and Annual Wormwood. It is known to be beneficial for respiratory congestion, infections, catarrh, and as a womb tonic. It has anti-cancer and anti-malarial properties and is effective against intestinal parasites. Constituent: Ketones/Lactones. Descriptor: Sedative, antispasmodic, mucolytic.

BALSAM of PERU, Wild: Peru (*Myroxylon balsamum*) – It is wonderful smelling but has some drawbacks when it comes to using it. It is black, gummy, and will stain anything it comes in contact with so use carefully. It works for infections, inflammation, bacteria, parasites, catarrh, as an antiseptic (pulmonary, urinary) and promotes epithelial cell growth. The epithelium is the cellular tissue covering surfaces, forming glands, and lining most cavities of the body. It is a diuretic, expectorant and stimulant. Beneficial for dry, chapped skin (use on skin diluted in carrier oil), eczema, diaper rashes, cracked nipples, sores, wounds, parasites (ringworm, itch mite, and eggs), scabies, fungus, chronic asthma, bronchitis (chronic and asthmatic), coughs, tuberculosis, and lessens mucus secretions.

Balsam of Peru assists rheumatism pain, stimulates the heart, increases blood pressure, is beneficial against the flu, colds, viral infections, cystitis (coli-bacillus), stress, and nervous tension. Found effective for scabies in dogs and cats by brushing it on the fur. It has a wonderful aroma everyone will enjoy, promotes feelings of safety, and of being nurtured. Constituent: Monoterpenes/Esters. Descriptor: Stimulates liver, aids digestion, tonic, decongestant and antispasmodic. Found in Peaceful Moments.

BASIL, Organically Grown: India (*Ocimum basilicum*) – GRAS – It has been known to help when used for inflammation, intestinal problems, respiratory ailments, repairing connective tissue, asthma, emphysema, bronchitis, chronic nasal catarrh, whooping cough, sinusitis, gout, rheumatism, muscular aches and pains, poor memory, mental fatigue, and loss of concentration. It is an insect repellent, beneficial when used for insect and snake bites and effective against wasp stings. It is beneficial against flu, colds, constipation, fainting, earache, gas, nausea, cramps, scanty periods, fevers, loss of smell and prostate problems.

Basil assists with hair growth and adds luster to dull hair. It is an acne skin tonic, effective against infectious disease, anxiety, depression, migraine, nervous tension, and stress. Basil is antiseptic and restorative as a stimulant for nerves and the adrenal cortex. It is beneficial for infections, spasms, as a heart tonic, stimulates blood flow, decongests veins and pulmonary arteries and promotes milk flow in nursing mothers. Aromatic influences: excellent aromatic nerve tonic, gives the mind strength, clears head, relieves intellectual fatigue, clarity, and eases "cold" feelings. Descriptor: Sedative, antispasmodic, expectorant, antiviral, antioxidant. Constituent: Ketones/Oxides. Found in Nerve Repair, Migraine Relief, and Focus.

BAY LEAF, Wild: Turkey (*Laurus nobilis*) (Laurel leaf) – GRAS – Bay Leaf has been helpful for flu, dyspepsia, gas, viral infections, and loss of appetite. The properties are digestive, stomachic, antiseptic, diuretic and a fungicidal. It is a tonic to the kidneys, liver, and reproductive system. Bay Leaf regulates scanty periods, urinary tuberculosis, and speeds delivery in childbirth.

It eases arthritis, ear and sinus infection, lowers blood pressure, beneficial for sprains, rheumatism, headaches, toothaches, and general aches and pains. For lymph swelling rub a few drops of Bay Leaf on the area. It assists anxiety, fears, and problems in expressing and manifesting possibilities, anti-depressant, psychosis, brings fire to one's life warming the emotions, assists all degenerative psychic pathologies, and gives confidence, awareness, and courage.

The ancient Greek and Romans used Bay leaves to crown their victors. It is wonderful to use in making soups and stews and **only one** drop is needed. It is excellent used in making stuffing and basting a turkey. Bay Leaf is relatively non-toxic but could be a skin irritant. Moderate use is recommended.

Several reports suggest it should not be used during pregnancy. Descriptor: Sedative, antispasmodic, antibiotic, antiseptic, expectorant, antioxidant, antifungal. Constituent: Ketone/Phenols/Oxides.

BAY/RUM, Wild: Jamaica *(Pimenta racemosa)* This Bay is much like the *Laurus nobilis*, it has a better smell, and works well for hair loss. Constituent: Eugenol/Other Alcohols. Descriptor: Analgesic, anticonvulsant.

BERGAMOT, Organically Grown: Italy *(Citrus aurantium)* – It has been helpful for acne, boils, cold sores, herpes infections, alleviating pain of shingles and chickenpox, oily complexion, excellent for psoriasis, scabies, and varicose ulcers. It is used for clearing excess mucus from the body, halitosis, mouth infections, tonsillitis, and loss of appetite. It assists cystitis, thrush, leucorrhea, colds, fevers, flu, is an antiseptic, and works well for infectious diseases, childhood diseases, and immune deficiency.

Bergamot assists anxiety, depression, stress, calms anger, and is refreshing, stimulating, uplifting, and gives self-confidence. It may assist during times of sadness or grieving and has been known to reopen the heart center so emotional wounds may heal. It restores joy, loving feelings, and the desire to give out to help others. It keeps the mind young and alert. Aromatic influence: may stabilize a person in a shaky emotional state. Diffused may assist in breaking the smoking habit. Constituent: Esters/Monoterpenes. Descriptor: Alkalizing (alterative), antispasmodic, stimulates liver, aids digestion. **NOTE:** The Bergamot, FCF, has the chemical that is phototoxic removed. Found in Hormone Balance, In The Moment, Love, Guardian, Magnify, Passion for Life, and Citrus Plus.

BIRCH BARK, Sweet Wild: USA *(Betula lenta)* It works well for many things but since it causes toxic build-up in the liver it is suggested to be used sparingly. It is excellent when used for inflammation, broken and bruised bones because of its high

cortisone-like properties. Other things you might use it for in small amounts are muscle and joint discomfort, gout, arthritis, cellulites, edema, poor circulation, rheumatism, cramps, and tendonitis. It is important to cleanse the liver often when using this copal. Aromatic influences: elevating and opening, increasing awareness in the sensory system. Constituent: Esters. Descriptor: Anti-inflammatory, antispasmodic. Found in Relief, Pain EZ, and Sport Pro.

BLACK CUMIN, Organically Grown: Egypt *(Nigella sativa)* – GRAS – In the Arab countries it is said, "Black Cumin heals every disease except for death." It is used as a digestive aid, an effective medicine for colds, headaches, toothaches, and infections. Because of its complex chemical structure (more than one hundred active ingredients) it has positive effects on the respiratory, circulatory, digestive, immune, and urinary systems of the body. Recent research has verified claims that Black Cumin strengthens and stabilizes the immune system and is effective in the treatment of asthma, allergies and other immune disorders as well as numerous skin conditions ranging from Rosacea to psoriasis.

Black Cumin has helped with bronchial spasm, spasmodic coughs, muscle pain, osteo-arthritis, and rheumatism, accumulation of fluid or toxins, poor circulation and lymphatic congestion. It is known to be useful for colic, mumps, glandular swelling, dyspepsia, flatulence, colitis, debility, constipation, frigidity, insomnia, migraine, nervous exhaustion, tiredness and lethargy. It is beneficial against hepatitis, hypothyroidism, normalizes menstrual cycles and testicular inflammation. Descriptor: Anti-inflammatory, antispasmodic. Constituent: Aldehydes/Monoterpenes. Found in Fortify, Freedom, Freedom Plus, and Rejuvenate.

BLACK PEPPER, Organically Grown: Madagascar *(Piper nigrum)* – GRAS – It assists in stimulating the endocrine system, gives energy, relieves pain, fights infections, reduces fevers, improves digestion and constipation. It is beneficial for muscle spasms, gas, urination, circulation, rheumatoid arthritis, inflammation, catarrhal and is an expectorant. Aromatic influences: motivates one into action when feeling "stuck," stimulates mental energy, feelings of courage and bravery, particularly about public speaking. Descriptor: Stimulates liver, aids digestion, decongestant, expectorant, and antioxidant. Constituent: Monoterpenes/Oxides. Found in Angel Assist, Freedom, Freedom Plus, Magnify, and Sport Pro.

BLUE TANSY, Organically Grown: Morocco
(Tanacetum anuum) – It is beneficial for bruises, asthma, hypertension, fevers, nervous tension, stress, neuritis, cramps, rheumatism, arthritis, emphysema, colds, and muscular rheumatism. It assists as a thymus stimulant, is beneficial against certain forms of leukemia, fights inflammation, spasms, and is a tonic. It may induce menstruation so avoid during pregnancy. Aromatic influences: eases anxiety, promote relaxation, gives patience, peace, very soothing, and calms worries. Constituent: Sesquiterpenes-Monoterpenes. Descriptor: Inflammation, stimulates liver, anti-lipic, aids digestion, decongestant. Found in True Blue, Peaceful Moments, Calming, Faith, Fortify, Break Thru, Confidence, and Serenity.

CAJEPUT, Organically Grown: Vietnam
(Melaleuca cajuputi) – GRAS – It is held in high regard in the Middle East and used for colds, headaches, throat infections, toothaches, sore and aching muscles, fever (cholera) and various skin problems. It is beneficial for chronic laryngitis, bronchitis, cystitis, rheumatism, oily skin, spots, arthritis, asthma, catarrh, coughs, sinusitis, flu, and viral infections. It is known to expel roundworms, and is beneficial to take the itch out of insect bites. Constituent: Oxides/Esters. Descriptor: Antioxidant, expectorant, alkalizing, antispasmodic.

CALAMUS: India (Acorus calamus) – It is a stimulating nerve antispasmodic, a general tonic to the mind rejuvenating the brain and nervous system. Calamus is used to promote cerebral circulation, to stimulate self-expression, and to help manage a wide range of symptoms in the head, including

neuralgia, epilepsy, memory loss, and shock. Found in Exodus.

CARDAMOM, Organically Grown: Guatemala
(Elettarria cardamomum) – GRAS – It has been used in traditional Chinese and Indian medicine for over 3000 years, especially for pulmonary disease, fever, digestive, and urinary complaints. Hippocrates recommended it for sciatica, coughs, abdominal pains, spasms, nervous disorders, urine retention, and bites of venomous creatures. Cardamom is beneficial for anorexia, loss of appetite, colic, cramps, dyspepsia, and gas, gripping pains, halitosis, heartburn, vomiting, mental fatigue, and nervous strain. It is alkalizing, antioxidant, and antispasmodic. Used in flavoring pastries, cookies, and cakes. Descriptor: Antioxidant, expectorant, alkalizing, antispasmodic. Constituent: Oxides/Esters. Found in Focus.

CARROT SEED, Organically Grown: India
(Daucus carota) – GRAS - The seeds are used to increase urine flow, for colic, kidney problems, infections, digestive disorders, and to promote menstruation. It has anti-septic properties that can prevent tetanus. It is beneficial for any skin infections such as sores, rashes, gangrene, psoriasis, and ulcers. When taken internally it is effective against infections of the throat, mouth, colon, stomach, intestines, urinary, and especially the whole respiratory system.

Carrot seed oil is effective in fighting other viral infections such as flu, mumps, cough, colds, and measles. It has the ability to detoxify the blood, tissues, muscles, and internal organs like the liver and kidneys. It can neutralize excess bile secreted from the liver and can help in cases of jaundice. It removes accumulations of toxins like uric acid from the blood, tissues, muscles and joints, thereby helping with edema, arthritis, grout, and rheumatism. Recent studies have shown it is beneficial in some forms of cancer, especially those of the mouth, throat, stomach, prostrate, and kidneys.
The anti-oxidants in carrot seeds repair all the damages done to your tissues by free radicals and

stop them from doing further harm. The anti-oxidants in carrot seeds are beneficial for wrinkles, joints, muscles, hair, eyes, macular degeneration, sexual weakness, weak digestion, and other related aging problems. Carrot seeds assist in dermatitis, eczema, revitalizing and toning, anemia, mature complexions, anorexia, liver congestion, and glandular problems. It is mild and has a soothing earthly aroma which is effective in relieving stress and anxiety. Descriptor: Sedative, relaxant, stimulant, inflammation, alkalizing, spasms, aids digestion, stimulates liver. Constituent: Alcohols/Esters/Monoterpenes. Found in Skin Care.

CASSIA Wild: India (Cinnamomum cassis) – Useful against colds, bronchitis pleurisy, rheumatism, tropical infections, and fevers. It stimulates both the digestion and circulation, and is beneficial for edema, diarrhea, dysentery, intestinal infections, gut parasites (amoebas, amoebic cysts), loss of appetite, and symptoms of poor circulation in the extremities. Cassia encourages effective peristaltic movements, reducing griping, and gas. Its strong antibacterial quality helps with pyorrhea, gum disease, adult intestinal toxemia, Candida infections and urinary infections. It is known to be effective for skin infections such as acne and boils. Found in Exodus.

CEDARWOOD, Wild: Himalaya (Cedrus deodara) – In India it is used effectively to cure ulcers, skin diseases, and repel mosquitoes. Known to control odors, respiratory infections, congestion, chronic bronchitis, coughs, catarrh, rheumatism, arthritis pain, sinusitis, and stimulates lymphatic circulation. It assists the immune system, arterial regeneration, wound healing, and boils. Cedarwood is antiseptic, assists urinary track infections (particularly cystitis and urethritis), simple water retention, tuberculosis, acne, dandruff, hair loss, dermatitis, psoriasis, oily skin, scalp, and hair.

It is beneficial for fungal infections, poisoning, stress-related conditions, meditation and clearing mental cobwebs. It assists in adding balance, and

control to our life regulating the nervous system and acts as a sedative in overcoming anger. Aromatic influence: calming, assists spirituality, and self-control. Descriptor: Inflammation, sedative, anti-lipic, antispasmodic. Constituent: Sesquiterpenes-Ketones. Found in Grounding, Bug Free, In The Moment, Mountain Retreat, Uplifting, DNA Repair, and Hair Support.

CELERY SEED, Organically Grown: India *(Apium graveolens)* – GRAS - May assist in decreasing puffy, red, water-logged skin, skin stains, spots, bronchitis, congestion, arthritis, gout pain, rheumatism, swollen glands, liver congestion, hemorrhoids, indigestion, bad breath, cystitis, gout, milk flow, menstruation, neuralgia, sciatica, and nervous disorders. It is beneficial for dissolving accumulated uric acid in joints and decreases toxin accumulation. Celery seeds assists lymphatic drainage, lowers blood pressure, balances glandular problems, assists in renal detoxification, increases urine flow, minimizes sexual problems, and is a sedative and tonic to the Central Nervous System for restful sleep. It may be used in soups, salads and sauces. It is thought best to avoid during pregnancy. Descriptor: Stimulates liver, digestion, tonic, anti-lipid, inflammatory. Constituent: Monoterps/Sesquiterps. Found in Slim & Trim.

CHAMOMILE, GERMAN, Organically Grown: Hungary *(Matricaria recutita)* – The yellow cone shaped flower contains the plant's medicinal properties and is beneficial for teething pain, earache, acne, eczema, dermatitis, sensitive skin, rashes, boils, burns, chilblains, inflammation, allergies, insect bites, hair care, bruises, cuts, wounds, inflamed joints, sprains, rheumatism, muscular pain, and neuralgia.

It is beneficial to use for indigestion, colic, diarrhea, nausea, menopausal problems, insomnia, nervous tension, migraines, stress related complaints, and neutralize allergies. Apply over the throat to assist in expressing your true feelings. Aromatic influence: the ability to relieve stress, tension, promotes peace, dispel anger, stabilize, and release emotions links to the past. Constituent: Oxides/Sesquiterp Alcohol. Descriptor: Expectorant, antioxidant, stimulator, alkalizing. Found in True Blue, Balance, Magnify, Break Thru, Serenity, and Vitality.

CHAMOMILE, ROMAN, Organic: England

(Anthemis nobilis) – GRAS – It is excellent for acne, dry itchy skin, dermatitis, eczema, psoriasis, hypersensitive skin, broken veins, inflammation, eases skin puffiness and strengthens the tissues. It is beneficial when used for boils, burns, cuts, allergies, and asthma caused by nervousness. It has analgesic action and eases arthritis, low back and muscle pain, rheumatism, sprains, and inflamed joints. It is beneficial for chronic infections, mouth ulcers, toothache, digestive complaints by soothing the stomach, relieves gastritis, diarrhea, ulcers, vomiting, colitis, assists irritable bowel syndrome, colic nausea, and intestinal parasites.

It stimulates production of white corpuscles and is beneficial to use before and after surgical procedures. It induces menstruation, eases painful difficult periods, regulates cycles, PMS, and irritability. It may be effective against anemia and jaundice. Aromatic influence: a relaxant, sedative, eases anxiety, worries, nervous system shock, tension, anger, fear, gives patience, peace, and calms the mind. Excellent made into an herb tea sweetened with stevia or honey. Descriptor: Alkalizing, anti-spasmodic, sedative, and stimulates liver. Constituent: Esters/Ketones/Monoterps. Found in Migraine Relief, Skin Care, Grateful, Faith, and Magnify.

CINNAMON BARK, Wild: Madagascar

(Cinnamomum zeylanicum) – GRAS – Here you want the true Cinnamon Bark. It assists circulation, lowering glucose, strengthens the heart, endocrine, and nervous systems. It is an immune stimulant and it has been found that viruses, bacteria, and fungus cannot live in this oil. Cinnamon Bark is used against parasites, typhoid, tropical infection, flu, colds, coughs, warts, rheumatism, and is a general all around maintenance oil, and general sexual

stimulant. It is a powerful purifier, enhances the action, and activity of the other oils.

Be careful you are not buying Cinnamon Leaf, which some suppliers label as Cinnamon since it has only very minimal benefits. Aromatic influences: May promote physical energy, psychic awareness, and increasing one's prosperity. Diffuse with caution and use in small amounts. It is best diffused mixed with other oils. **Caution when using Cinnamon Bark:** always dilute with carrier oil because the high phenol properties make it hot and will burn the skin. Constituent: Aldehydes-Phenols. Descriptor: Alkalizing, tonic, antibiotic, antiseptic. Found in Hormone Balance, Meditation, Cinnamon Blend, Exodus, First Aid, Prosperity, DNA Repair, Joyful, Rejuvenate, Slim & Trim, and Spice Traders.

CITRONELLA, Organically Grown: India

(Cymbopogon winterianus) – It has been used for its medicinal value in many cultures for fevers, intestinal parasites, digestive and menstrual problems, as a stimulant, insect repellent, and room deodorizer. Citronella is beneficial for oily skin and hair, excessive perspiration, colds, flu, inflammation, rheumatism and arthritis pain, minor infections, fatigue, headaches, migraines, stress, and nervous related conditions. Descriptor: Alkalizing, tonic, antibiotic, antiseptic. Constituent: Aldehydes-Phenols. Found in Bug Free, Passion for Life, Purify, and Serenity.

CLARY SAGE, Organic: Bulgaria (Salvia sclarea)

– It has been beneficial in regulating cells, hormonal imbalance, menstrual cramps by minimizing the pain, menopause problems, PMS, itching, and irritation of herpes. It assists with Candida outbreaks, infections, exhaustion, sore throat, nerves, mental strain, hostility, bronchitis, cholesterol, debility, genitals, hemorrhoids, frigidity, seborrhea, hair loss, scalp massage, acne and has been found to be extremely good for the skin. It is an antispasmodic that has been used to soothe asthma attacks, is used for blood pressure, hyperactivity, claustrophobia, and nightmares.

Clary Sage is a sedative and known to stimulate contractions in the last stages of childbirth. It strengthens the immune system, is beneficial to use in times of personal challenges or change, especially when there is external stress and pressure such as in a mid-life crisis. Aromatic influence: very calming, may enhance the dream state, and bring about a feeling of euphoria. Constituent: Esters/Mono Sesquiterps. Descriptor: Alkalizing, stimulates liver, inflammation, spasms, sedative. Found in Angel Assist, Support, and Hormone Balance.

CLOVE BUD, Organically Grown: Madagascar
(*Eugenia caryophyllata*) – GRAS - May assist the respiratory system, toothaches, pain, sore throat (2 drops in ½ c. water and gargle), infectious diseases (formerly used against the plague), infected wounds, memory deficiency, and impotence. It is an antiseptic and beneficial for inflammation, viruses, bacteria, fungus, tumors, and parasites assisting with athlete's foot, arthritis, rheumatism, and sprains.

Clove Bud is beneficial for colic, nausea, colds, flu, cancer, Hodgkin's, dental infections, virus of the nerves (MS), cystitis, diarrhea, amoebic dysentery, viral hepatitis, bacterial colitis, cholera, sinusitis, tuberculosis, hypertension, thyroid dysfunction, and fatigue. Aromatic influences: sense of healing, improved memory, protection, and courage. Constituent: Phenols/Esters. Descriptor: Antibiotic, antiseptic/alkalizing, antispasmodic, analgesic. Found in Relief, Spice Traders, Gentle Healer, Sports Pro, Fortify, Prosperity, Soothing Relief, and Rejuvenate. **Caution:** Insist on only Clove Bud; not the whole Clove plant.

COPAIBA BALSAM, Wild: (*Copaifera officinalis*) It is very high in sesquiterpenes, is a powerful anti-inflammatory, anti-bacterial, disinfectant (urinary and pulmonary), and diuretic. It assists with colds, chills, coughs, bronchitis, catarrh, and inflammation of the mucus membranes. It is beneficial with lymphatic flow, intestinal infections, eases vomiting, diarrhea, nervous tension, stress problems, and anxiety. Found in Soothing Relief.

CORIANDER, Organically Grown: Russia
(*Coriandrum sativum*) – GRAS - Beneficial for stretch marks and scars, arthritis, rheumatism, stiffness, gout, muscle aches and pains, intestinal spasm, accumulation of fluids or toxins, and increase circulation. It assists colds, flu, infectious diseases, measles, colic, anorexia, hiccups, diarrhea, gastritis, dyspepsia, nausea, piles, impotence, frigidity, infertility, has estrogen-like properties, postpartum care (depression), fear, migraine, nervous exhaustion, gentle mental stimulant for a bad memory, dizziness, and shock. Constituent: Aldehydes. Descriptor: Alkalizing, calming, anti-inflammatory, anti-febrile.

CUCUMBER SEED, Organically Grown: India
(*Cucumis sativus*) – *GRAS* – The oil is obtained from the clean dried seeds and is rich in important nutrients like Sodium, Fluorine, Chlorine, Potassium, and Magnesium. It can be effective in treating dry skin, eczema, psoriasis, sunburns, wrinkles, stretch marks, damaged hair, and brittle nails. This oil is a vital source of proteolytic enzymes, vitamin C, B1 that helps to revitalize, and detoxify the skin.

It has a cooling effect that works on your skin taking care of its problems from blackheads, eruptions, acne, and puffiness around the eyes. It assists in making the external skin soft and supple. It builds elasticity of naturally curly hair, keeping it strong, and preventing annoying breakage caused by weak, chemical, and/or heat damaged hair. The natural silica in the seed encourages new hair growth and helps to reduce the chances of hair loss. It helps healing of many illnesses including lung, stomach, and chest problems, gout, arthritis, and tapeworms.

The detoxifying effects of the Cucumber helps rid the skin of dirt and oil helping clear up blemishes. A little dash of Cucumber in a face mask or freshening gel and your skin starts glowing like never before. To make a good skin cleansing mixture add: Aloe Vera, Olive oil, and Cucumber together to cleanse the face night and morning. Mixing a few drops of Cucumber and one tablespoon of olive oil to gently massage your body will gradually reduce your stress or simply apply Cucumber oil on the temples offers amazing results. For burns add a few drops of Cucumber with Lavender before applying it to the burn. This highly moisturizing oil can be used in a wide range of applications including soaps, creams, and lotions. Descriptor: Anti-Aging, Anti-oxidant, and sedative. Constituent: Linoleic and Oleic Acid. Found in Skin Care.

CUMIN, Organically Grown: Turkey (*Cuminum cyminum*) – GRAS – It is an anti-oxidant, antiseptic, antispasmodic, and thyroid stimulant. It assists with asthma, bronchial spasm, muscle pain, spasmodic coughs, osteo-arthritis, and rheumatism. It is beneficial for lymphatic congestion, glandular swelling, mumps, the accumulation of fluid or toxins, poor circulation, inflammation, colic, colitis, assists hypo-thyroidism, indigestion, constipation, useful in hepatitis, increases thyroid function, frigidity, impotence (said to increase desire and fertility in males), eases testicular inflammation, normalizes menstrual cycle, and increases lactation. Used for debility, migraine, nervous exhaustion, tiredness, insomnia, and lethargy. Could possibly be phototoxic so avoid the direct sun on areas where the oils are applied. Descriptor: Alkalizing, calming, anti-inflammatory, anti-febrile, stimulates liver. Constituent: Aldehydes/Monoterpenes.

CYPRESS, Organically Grown: India (*Cupressus sempervirens*) – It improves circulation throughout the lungs and body, strengthens blood capillary walls, and decreases any excessive flow of fluids whether a runny nose, diarrhea, excessive menstrual flow or perspiration. It is beneficial for varicose veins, edema, cellulites, decongests the lymphatic, and prostate. Cypress is beneficial for pancreas insufficiency, gut infections, asthma, sluggish intestines, pulmonary tuberculosis, pyorrhea, pleurisy, insomnia, rheumatism, arthritis, bronchitis, whooping cough, and eliminates mucus.

Cypress stops bleeding gums or cuts, purifies blood, stimulates the immune system, tightens tissues, hemorrhoids - both internal and external, cramps,

menopausal problems acting as a female hormone stimulant, lack of concentration, stress, nervous tension and a general healer. It assists with transition or changing course in life. It is comforting and strengthening in times of death or divorce, uplifting, and fortifying. Use Cypress when there is sexual preoccupation or uncontrolled crying and talking. It gives energy and removes psychic blocks (purifies, cleans psychically and physically). It assists when used with lemon for young children deprived of parental affection and protection.

Aromatic influences: strengthens, eases the feeling of loss, creates a feeling of security and grounding, and heals emotions. Descriptor: Stimulates liver, anti-inflammatory, anti-lipic, antibiotic, and antiseptic. Constituent: Monoterpenes/Sesquiterpenes-Phenols. Found in Angel Assist, DNA Repair, Vision, Break Thru, Relief, Circle of Life, Toning, and Prosperity.

DILL SEED, Organically Grown: India (*Anethum graveolens*) – GRAS – It lowers glucose levels by normalizing insulin levels and supporting pancreatic functions. It assists colic, bronchial catarrh, eases congestion, vomiting, dry heaves, liver deficiencies, hiccups, indigestion, and promotes milk flow in nursing mothers. It is beneficial for bacteria, catarrh, spasms, parasites, is antiseptic, and anticoagulant (blood thinner). It assists with coronary thrombosis risk and calms the stomach. Descriptor: Sedative, antispasmodic, stimulates liver, anticoagulant. Constituent: Ketones/Monoterpenes/Courmarins.

ELEMI, Organically Grown: Philippines (*Canarium luzonicum*) – Elemi gum was traditionally used by the Egyptians for the embalming process. It is antiviral, antiseptic, fungicidal, general regulatory tonic (fortifying), and stimulant for stomach and glands. It is beneficial for aged skin, infected cuts, wounds, wrinkles, inflammation, chronic conditions, fungal growths, and gangrene conditions. Generally it fortifies the body and stimulating the thymus gland. It is beneficial for bronchitis, coughs, controls excess mucus, eases congestion, rejuvenates and strengthens the immune system, particularly at the start of an illness. Elemi is beneficial for diarrhea, various ulcers, spasmodic intestinal colitis, amoebic infections, nervous exhaustion, and stress.

There may be a possible cross sensitivity to Balsam of Peru. Aromatic influences: grounding and joyous, instills peace, centering, balances both the upper and lower chakras, visualization, helps reach deep hidden emotions which would make it good to use with Trauma-Gone. Elemi is closely related to the Myrrh and Frankincense trees. Descriptor: Stimulates liver, aids digestion, decongestant, anti-inflammatory, antispasmodic. Constituent: Monoterpenes/Sesquiterpenes. Found in Baby Soft, Break Thru, and DNA Repair.

EUCALYPTUS CITRIODORA, Wild: India

(Eucalyptus citriodora) – This eucalyptus is a powerful antiseptic and beneficial for athlete's foot, fungal infections, insecticide, dandruff, herpes, sores, asthma, laryngitis, sore throat, colds, fevers, and infectious skin conditions such as chickenpox. It assists arthritis, rheumatoid arthritis, rheumatism, muscle and joint aches and pains, injuries, and sprains. It assists hypertension, lowers blood pressure, is a recovery support after a heart attack, and assists in recuperating from long illness. It is soothing, calming, eases shingle pain, increases urine flow, and is a urinary antiseptic. It is a powerful antispasmodic, anti-inflammatory, deodorant, expectorant, fungicidal, insect repellant, and purifier. Aromatic influences: promotes health, well-being, purification, and healing. Diffusing helps stop the spread of infection. Constituent: Aldehydes-Monoterpenes. Descriptor: Expectorant stimulates liver. Found in Breathe EZ and Circle of Life.

EUCALYPTUS GLOBULUS, Wild: India

(Eucalyptus globulus) – It is analgesic, fights fungus (Candida), bacteria (strong action), microbes (staph, strep, coli, typhus), spasms, viruses, infections, makes a good deodorant, and is an immune stimulant. Choose over Eucalyptus citriodora when there is phlegm pattern-predominance of cold, white,

watery mucus in lungs, and sinuses, joints may be affected, and tongue thick with sticky white coat. It is beneficial for cuts, lice, insect bites, repellant, increases respiratory metabolism of skin cells (oxygen discharge, carbon dioxide intake), and oxygenates the skin. It has a regenerative effect on pulmonary tissue, aids chronic bronchitis, tuberculosis, pulmonary gangrene, diphtheria, catarrh, coughs, sinusitis, flu, throat infections, pneumonia, and deep lung infections.

It is beneficial for muscle aches and pains, arthritis, poor circulation, and swollen glands (infections). Assists in genito-urinary infections, inflammation (especially E. coli), headaches, concentration, and clears the head. It assists hemorrhages, epidemics (chickenpox, measles, and cholera), fevers, malaria, typhus, roseola, and an immune stimulant. Aromatic influences: promotes health, purification, well-being, and healing. Diffusing helps stop the spread of infection. **Caution:** This oil should **never** be taken internally; it may be fatal. A death of a child was reported after ingesting 5 mls. Avoid applying near infants' nostrils because of risk of spasm due to cooling effect on the respiratory system. Descriptor: Expectorant, alkalizing, antioxidant, stimulates liver. Constituent: Oxides/Monoterpenes/Aldehydes. Found in Breathe EZ and Vision.

EUCALYPTUS RADIATA, Organic: Australia

(Eucalyptus radiata) – GRAS – Known to be beneficial for sinus problems, asthma, bronchitis, catarrh, mouth infections, coughs, and sore throat. It fights infections, viruses, inflammation, bacteria, catarrh, and is an expectorant. This chemotype is better suited for long term use for chronic respiratory conditions and best suited for viral or bacteria infections. It is safe to inhale directly to lessen cough reflexes.

Choose Eucalyptus radiata over Eucalyptus globulus when infections are higher in the chest. It eases endometriosis inflammation, arthritis (especially rheumatoid arthritis), muscle aches, pains, injuries, sprains, flu, cold, fevers, leucorrhea, cystitis, headaches, nervous exhaustion, neuralgia, and sciatica. Aromatic influences: promotes health, well-being, purification, and healing. Constituent: Oxides/Monoterpenes-Aldehydes. Descriptor: Expectorant, antioxidant, stimulates liver, alkalizing. Found in Breathe EZ, Rejuvenate, Bug Free, and Spice Traders.

FENNEL SEED, Sweet, Organically Grown: Turkey (*Foeniculum vulgare Miller*) – GRAS – It supports the digestive function, assists the liver in producing enzymes, balances hormones, relieves emotional stress, increases lactation and supports the body in reducing PMS and menopausal symptoms. Fennel assists the liver, kidneys, spleen, urinary stones, gout, cystitis, gas, intestinal spasms, vomiting, intestinal parasites, and diabetes. It fights inflammation, infections, clears excess mucus, and acts as a diuretic. Assists with urinary infections, asthma, rheumatism, bronchitis, constipation, eye problems, hiccups, and improves overall body function. It is beneficial for bruises, cellulites, gums, halitosis, mouth, nausea, obesity, toxin build-up, and water retention.

Fennel restores moisture to dry and dehydrated skin and restores muscle tone. Regularly massaging on the breasts is said to keep them firm and attractive. It is used in Europe for its detoxifying action in treatment of alcohol and drug abuse and is said to counteract alcohol poisoning. Fennel seed assists the reproductive system. Aromatic influences: longevity, courage, and purification. Descriptor: Antispasmodic, sedative, adaptogenic, stimulates liver. Constituent: Phenolpropanes/Monoterpenes-Ketones. Found in Tummy Rub and Toning.

FIR NEEDLE, Wild: Austria (*Abies alba*) – Assists acute chronic bronchitis, chills, coughs, flu, sinusitis, arthritis, muscular aches and pain, rheumatism, colds, and fevers. It is grounding, immune stimulating, antiseptic, anti-catarrhal, benefits the nervous system, is good for debility, asthenia tension, and stress. It acts as a sedative yet is elevating to the mind. Aromatic influences: fights airborne germs and bacteria when diffused.

Constituent: Monoterpenes/Esters. Descriptor: Stimulate liver, antispasmodic, aid digestion, tonic alkalizing. Found in Meditation, Mountain Retreat, and Joyful.

FRANKINCENSE, Wild: Somalia and India (*Boswellia carterii*) – GRAS – The therapeutic quality of both types of Frankincense are basically the same. The India Frankincense is used in the Ayurvedic medicine and has a very unique smell that most people would not associate with Frankincense. It is an incredible immune system builder, beneficial for catarrhal, inflammation, tumors, asthma, bronchitis, tuberculosis, digestive disorders, and lymph congestion, infections, reproductive and urinary difficulties.

Frankincense is used for skin ulcers, scars and blemishes, balances oily skin, dry and mature complexions, smooths out wrinkles, and is an antiseptic tonic for all skin types. A diluted blend of Frankincense rubbed into the abdomen regularly during pregnancy prevents stretch marks. It assists laryngitis, colds, flu, fevers, anxiety, nightmares, fear of the future, nervous tension, and stress-related conditions. It tones the uterus and relieves uterine hemorrhaging and heavy menstrual flow, eases labor pains, and decreases postnatal depression.

It fortifies the mind, assists indecision, depression, eliminates blocked personal growth, and tension. It heals emotional wounds, stabilizes and centers the emotions, and focuses energy. It slows breathing, producing a calm, soothing, elevated mental state, brings peace, strengthens beliefs, assists divine connections, cleans the aura, and psychic planes. Because it contains sesquiterpenes this enables it to go beyond the blood brain barrier to assist in increasing oxygen around the pineal and pituitary glands.

Aromatic influences: recognized for increasing spiritual awareness and meditation. Descriptor: Stimulates liver, aids digestion, anti-lipic, anti-inflammatory, sedative, and antispasmodic.

Constituent: Monoterpenes/Sesquiterpenes-Ketones/Oxides. Found in Balance, Confidence, Exodus, Fortify, Vision, Grounding, Magnify, Meditation, Mountain Retreat, Passion for Life, Prosperity, Rejuvenate, Joyful, DNA Repair, Peaceful Moments, Skin Care, and Utopia.

GALBANUM, Organically Grown: Afghanistan, Hydro-distilled *(Ferula galbaniaflua)* – GRAS – It is said to have been a favorite oil of Moses. It has its own distinct smell. It has been beneficial for abscesses, acne, boils, cuts, inflammation, heals scar tissue, tones skin, is beneficial for wrinkles, and mature skin. It is analgesic, antiseptic, fights microbes and viruses, is beneficial for circulation, asthma, bronchitis, chronic coughs, cramps, rheumatism, muscular aches and pains, indigestion and nervous tension. Galbanum is a diuretic, restorative, tonic, and strengthens the whole system. Alone its frequency is low, but when combined with other copals such as Frankincense or Sandalwood, the frequency changes drastically. Descriptor: Stimulates liver, aids digestion, decongestant, alkalizing, anticoagulant, sedating. Constituent: Monoterpenes/Esters/Courmarins. Found in Exodus and Overcome.

GERANIUM, Organically Grown: Egypt *(Pelargonium graveolens)* **and GERANIUM BOURBON, Rose Geranium: Madagascar** *(Pelargonium roseum)* – GRAS - The benefits of the two are similar with the rose geranium having a rosy smell and is more expensive. Some women love using rose geranium for hot flashes better than progesterone cream. Both Geraniums have been beneficial for acne, dermatitis, eczema, broken capillaries, cellular regeneration, and wound healing - especially after facial or plastic surgery. They balance all gland secretion for oily, congested and mature skin, assists with cellulite, sore throat, burns, tonsillitis, asthma, mucus, bruises, rheumatism, circulation, hemorrhoids, gastritis, itching, immune stimulation, liver tonic, jaundice, colitis, and sterility. Rub on the back of both partners for infertility. Both Geraniums are effective for hormonal disturbances, PMS, menopause, and engorged breasts. They

contain anticoagulant properties and may stimulate the lymphatic system.

Geranium is neuro-balancing, a sedative, reduces stress, anti-depressant, soothes anxiety, assists with diarrhea, ulcers, urinary stones, bleeding, edema, tones and tightens tissues, diabetes, lowers blood sugar levels, hemorrhoids, gallbladder, fights infection, fungus, lice and ringworm, and cleans the digestive system of mucus. It assists the adrenal glands is consoling, beneficial for overcoming acute fear, hurt, extreme moodiness, depression, and in raising self-esteem.

For abuse issues apply over the abdomen and in an emotional crisis use it in a full body massage. Aromatic influence: assists in letting go of the negative past, assists one to overcome fear of speaking, eases the anxiety and tension of mentally and physically demanding days. Descriptor: Stimulates liver, aids digestion, decongestant, alkalizing, spasms, sedative, anticoagulant. Constituent: Monoterpenes/Esters-Ketones. **Caution:** Some say this oil should be avoided in early pregnancy. Geranium is found in Angel Assist, Baby Soft, Guardian, Balance, Utopia, and Vitality. Rose Geranium is found in Break Thru, Love, Toning, and Passion for Life.

GINGER ROOT, Organically Grown: India *(Zingiber officinale)* – GRAS – It is beneficial for bruises, sores, sprains, strains, carbuncles, broken bones, muscular aches and pains, cramps, arthritis, poor circulation, rheumatism, catarrh, chronic bronchitis, congestion, cough, colds, chills, flu, fever, sinusitis, sore throat, tonsillitis, swollen glands, and dries excess mucus. It regulates moisture reducing the drainage of a runny nose and eases respiratory infections. Ginger assists with memory, gas, digestion, and diarrhea, loss of appetite, colic, nausea, motion sickness, morning sickness, infections, fatigue, tiredness, contagious diseases, nervous exhausting, and alcoholism. It is stimulating but grounding, warms cold emotions, and sharpens senses (psychic sponge). Use for over sensitivity and protection. Aromatic influences: enhances physical energy, money, and courage. It sharpens the senses, improves memory, and assists in recall. Constituent: Sesquiterpenes/Monoterpenes. Descriptor: Anti-inflammatory, toxic, stimulates liver, aids digestion, decongestant. Found in Tummy Rub, Slim & Trim, Circle of Life, Dreamtime, Fortify, Rejuvenate, and Spice Traders.

GRAPEFRUIT, Pink and White, Organic: USA Pressed Peel (Citrus paradisi) – GRAS – The pink grapefruit smells better but the white has more detoxifying effects when used internally for digestion, eases water retention, increases urine flow, stimulates the gallbladder, liver tonic, useful in anorexia, bulimia, and regulates body weight if used regularly. It assists athlete's foot, acne, oily skin, cellulite, tones congested skin, tightens skin, airborne disinfectant when diffused, eases muscle fatigue, stiffness, increases circulation, stimulates the lymphatic system, detoxifies, cold, chills, and flu.

Grapefruit may assist hair growth and is beneficial for nervous exhaustion, jet lag, performance stress, headaches, PMS, drug and alcohol withdrawal, depression, and self-doubt. Aromatic influences: uplifting, gives confidence, and prevents one from drowning in one's own negativity. Constituents: Monoterpenes-Aldehydes. Descriptor: Stimulates liver, aids digestion, alkalizing, anti-inflammatory, and antiseptic. Found in Peacemaker, Citrus Plus, Peaceful Moments, and Slim & Trim.

HELICHRYSUM, Organic: Madagascar
(Helichrysum gymnocephalum) – This species is much less expensive. It is anti-inflammatory, analgesic, and antiseptic. It is used for cuts, wounds, bruises, ulcers, herpes, rheumatism, gingivitis, pyorrhea, gastritis, sore throat, and typhoid fever. It induces menstruation, assists painful menstruation and headaches, and induces milk flow. Descriptor: Alkalizing, antispasmodic, tonic, calming/sedative, inflammation. Constituent: Esters/Ketones-Sesquiterpenes. Found in Relief, True Blue, and Migraine Relief.

HELICHRYSUM: Organically Grown: Croatia
(Helichrysum italicum) – This species is extremely beneficial for any nerve problem and is an excellent pain reliever. It has been used for hearing problems caused by nerve damage with good results. Also beneficial when used against allergic conditions, fungus, bacteria, infections, viruses, inflammation (properties that reduce inflammation exceed those of any other essential oil), hematoma (swelling or tumor full of diffused blood), and a powerful anticoagulant. It has virtually unlimited value in treating dermatitis, eczema, psoriasis, acne, scaring, sunburns, broken veins, stimulates the regeneration of new cells, stretch marks, and spots.

Helichrysum italicum assists muscular aches and pains, bruises, sprains, rheumatism, respiratory conditions, sinus infection, whooping cough, nerves, spleen, headaches, and pulmonary spasms. It assists in detoxifying, blood cleansing, stomach cramps, phlebitis, hypo-cholesterol, known to help stimulate the liver cell function, viral colitis, gallbladder infection, pancreas stimulant, lymph drainage, sciatica, and connective tissue repair (repairing nerve endings). It may assist in activating the right side of the brain, help with depression, stress, visualization, and personal growth.

Aromatic influences: enhances the subconscious and is uplifting. When we get angry, lock ourselves up inside, or won't forgive trespasses, we create barriers that keep us from going forward in our lives. Mix equal parts with Rose to unite head and heart. Constituent: Esters/Ketones-Sesquiterpenes. Descriptor: Promotes new cell growth, alkalizing, antispasmodic, anti-inflammatory tonic, calming. Found in Soothing Relief, Circle of Life, Gentle Healer, Freedom, Freedom Plus, Vision, Passion for Life, Migraine Relief, Nerve Repair, DNA Repair, Utopia, and Rejuvenate.

HOLY BASIL, Organically Grown: India (Ocimum sanctum) – This is capable of rejuvenating the system quickly. It is anti-allergic, antispasmodic, fights infections, viruses, fungus, and bacteria. It enhances immunity, metabolic functions, reduces stress, beneficial for asthma, diabetes, coughs, mild upper respiratory infections, and indigestion.

It has been used in the treatment of ringworm, malaria, cholera, constipation, vomiting, catarrh, ear infections, dysentery, fever, nerves, and protects against stress induced ulcers. It is a powerful mosquito repellent, deodorant, cardio tonic, blood purifier. Dilute when used for skin disorders. Constituent: Eugenol/Monoterpenes. Descriptor: Antispasmodic, aids pancreas, sedative, aids digestion. Found in Focus, Fortify, Hair Support, Passion for Life, and Magnify.

HYSSOP, Wild: Spain *(Hyssop decumbens)* – It is one of the bitter herbs mentioned in the Bible used to purify the temple. It is a symbol of spiritual cleansing. It helps prevent colds, flu, strengthens the lungs, benefits poor vitality, breathlessness, immune deficiency, stimulates and warms the digestion, and may be used for appetite loss, abdominal bloating, slow digestion, and works to fight infection. Its effect on the nervous system and mind is a distinctly invigorating one and is recommended for poor concentration, mental fatigue, and chronic nervous debility.

According to Oriental Medicine, it protects both physically and psychologically and was once considered the "Herb of Protection" since it was thought to defend the individual and their home from negative influences. It benefits the type of person who is easily affected by other's moods and emotions, and who, as a result, quickly absorbs any tension in the environment. It helps to purge confused thoughts and negative emotions, which leads to greater spiritual insight and generosity.

Other benefits of Hyssop are to discharge toxins, stimulate and decongest the liver, clear lungs, open up the respiratory system, and normalize blood pressure. It assists against bronchitis, colic, fatigue, colds, sore throat, dermatitis, bruises, gout, nervous tension, arthritis, pulmonary inflammation, and

rheumatism. It is beneficial for hepatitis, assists nervous depression, anxiety, intestinal parasites, cystitis, regulates lipid metabolism. Use in moderation, only four or five drops in a massage, as it is very hot and stimulating by nature. Constituent: Oxides-Monoterpenes/ Sesquiterps. Descriptor: Expectorant, antioxidant, stimulates liver, aids digestion, anti-inflammatory, alkalizing, tonic, antispasmodic. Found in Balance, Circle of Life, Exodus, Fortify, Guardian, and DNA Repair.

JASMINE, Organically Grown, Absolute: India *(Jasminum grandiflorum)* – This jasmine blooms during the day and is considered the fun loving fragrance. It has benefited stress, hoarseness, laryngitis, menstrual problems, lethargy (abnormal drowsiness), inflammation, nervous exhaustion, impotence, frigidity, uterine disorders, and all types of skin problems. It assists low self-confidence, anxiety, apathy, depression, pessimism, dispels fear, paranoia, indifference, listlessness, and emotional suffering. It is best used near the end of pregnancy because it has been known to ease labor pains, encourage contractions, assist the expulsion of the afterbirth, and overall recovery from giving birth. It relieves postnatal depression, assists in stimulating milk production, and tones the uterus.

Jasmine may strengthen the male reproductive system and relieve discomfort of an enlarged prostate gland. Aromatic influences: may spur creativity, inspire artistic expression, awaken intuition, arouse an appreciation of beauty in the world, and dissolve emotional blocks that hinder personal growth. **Caution:** Since it can stimulate menstruation, avoided using during pregnancy until childbirth is imminent. Descriptor: Stimulant, tonic, alkalizing, sedative, antispasmodic. Constituent: Alcohols-Esters/Ketones. Found in Dreamtime, In The Moment, Jasmine Blend, Uplifting, and Passion for Life.

JUNIPER BERRY, Wild: Nepal *(Juniperus communis)* – GRAS – It helps in detoxifying and cleaning any kind of skin inflammation, skin ulcers, dermatitis, psoriasis, oily complexions, acne, eczema, a skin toner, and antiseptic. It is beneficial for hair loss, hemorrhoids, obesity, liver, kidney, urinary infections and bladder problems. The tree has been burned in many parts of the world to fight the spread of plagues, epidemics, and contagious diseases.

Juniper berry is beneficial for ulcers, respiratory problems, arthritis, bruises, infections, coughs, diuretic, cellulite, regulating menstrual cycle, cramps, and rheumatism. It is a local stimulant making it a good to use in a massage. It is used for anxiety, stress, nervous tension, clearing mental clutter and confusion, neutralizing negative exhausted emotions, imparting a feeling of emotional cleanliness. Aromatic influences: health, love, and peace. Best to use before meditation since it clears negative energy from the room. **Caution:** This is another essential oil you will need to check to make sure you are getting the berry. Descriptor: Stimulates liver, aids digestion, anti-inflammatory, antispasmodic, alkalizing, anti-febrile. Constituent: Monoterpenes/Sesquiterpenes-Aldehydes. Found in Fortify and Tummy Rub.

LAVENDER, Organically Grown: Hungary

(Lavandula angustifolia) –GRAS – This species is said to have a finer scent and is commonly grown in higher altitudes so it contains more esters. It is known to blend well with all essential oils and is considered one of the universal oils. When in doubt, Lavender is the one to use. It is beneficial used for spasms, infections, bacteria, inflammation, excellent for skin conditions, increases cell growth, and by applying to a wound or before having an operation, may assist the skin to heal and rejuvenate. It is beneficial for acne, burns, sunburn, stretch marks, minimizing scarring, boils, bruises, wounds, lice, ringworm, dermatitis, diaper rash, eczema, thrush, cankers, mouth abscess, tonsillitis, hair loss, and dandruff.

Lavender assists arthritis, rheumatism, sciatica, muscular aches and pains, colic, abdominal cramps, dyspepsia, indigestion, nausea, gas, lowering blood pressure, and fluid retention. It is excellent for insomnia, tachycardia, phlebitis, allergies, asthma, fainting, cuts, headaches, hysteria, stings, and insect bites. It assists in eliminating waste through the lymphatic system, herpes, pre-menstrual and menopausal problems, ulcers, athlete's foot, earache, flu, chronic fatigue syndrome, and boosts immunity. Food cravings are often a reaction to stress. So when you're feeling tense, relax your mind with a few drops of lavender massaged into your temples and your solar plexus for a reminder to relax, and breathe deeply.

Lavender balances extremes in emotions, irritability, moodiness, fear, change, insecurity, inner child, PMS, restlessness, depression, shock, vertigo, and nerves. When gallstones cause gallbladder spasms, place a few drops of Lavender in a hot tub of water and soak your whole body until the water cools or the spasms pass. A few drops of Lavender oil added to your body lotion can be a source of anxiety preventing aromatherapy all day long.

Aromatic influences: consciousness, health, love, and peace. When angry massage the solar plexus with lavender. It calm emotional extremes and aid deep trance, and everyday spirituality – balance higher and lower chakras. Descriptor: Sedative, tonic, antispasmodic, anticoagulant, alkalizing, calming. Constituent: Ketones/Esters. Found in Bug Free, Vision, Break Thru, First Aid, Faith, Skin Care, Grounding, Magnify, Rejuvenate, Balance, Utopia, Serenity, Migraine Relief, and Toning.

LEMON, Organic USA Pressed Peel: (Citrus limonum) – GRAS – Lemon pressed peel has many therapeutic properties but has a very short shelf life of about three years. It is beneficial to add a few drops to your water to assist the digestive system including the liver to go to work. It cleanses the lymphatic system, is stimulating to the brain, clears thoughts, helps concentration, and fights infectious diseases. It is beneficial for mouth ulcers, colds, flu, herpes, throat infection, asthma, bronchitis, anemia, heart-burn, varicose veins, tightens blood vessels,

rheumatism, arthritis, gallstones, dyspepsia, and gout. Lemon is used for acne, uterine infections, intestinal parasites, brittle nails, boils, warts, corns, gland stimulation and purification, cellulite, high blood pressure, stops nose bleeds, poor circulation, and reduces fevers. It is an air disinfectant, astringent, antiseptic, and stimulates the immune system in the formation of red and white blood cells. Lemon assists with debility, anxiety, apathy, nervous conditions, emotional clarity, awareness, brings joy, relieves touchiness, grudges, resentment, focus, and concentration.

If you are feeling queasy just open a bottle of Lemon oil and smell the clean, fresh citrus scent. It is known to promote spiritual and psychic awareness, supports the connection between spirit (consciousness) and soul, and beneficial when used for conflict in thoughts, and intellect. Aromatic influences are health, healing, physical energy, and purification. Excellent made into an herb tea sweetened with stevia or honey. Constituent: Monoterpenes/Aldehydes. Descriptor: Stimulates liver, aids in digestion, anti-inflammatory, alkalizing. Found in Hormone Balance, Rejuvenate, Love, In The Moment, Magnify, Citrus Plus, Balance, Prosperity, Slim & Trim, Spice Traders, and Soothing Relief.

LEMONGRASS, Wild: Nepal (*Cymbopogon citratus*) – GRAS – It stimulates the digestion and liver, regulates the Para-sympathetic system, strengthens vascular walls, and regenerates connective tissue. It fights fungus, is an immune stimulant, clears infections, repairs ligaments, improves eyesight and lymphatic drainage. Lemongrass is beneficial for bladder infection, kidney disorders, fluid retention, edema, varicose veins, and excessive perspiration, as an insect repellent against fleas, lice, and ticks.

It opens the pores, tones tissue and muscles, aids poor circulation, and stress. Aromatic influences: purification, psychic awareness, and calming. Descriptor: Alkalizing, anti-inflammatory, aids

digestion, stimulates liver, decongestant. Constituent: Aldehydes-Monoterpenes. Found in Freedom Plus, Purify, Pain EZ, Vision, Bug Off, Rejuvenate, and Toning.

LIME, Organically Grown: Mexico Distilled (*Citrus aurantifolia*) – Lime is often used indiscriminately in place of Lemon with which it shares many qualities. It is useful for viral infections, eases inflammation, fevers, flu, cough, cold congestion, muscle tonic, spasms, sore throat, liver pain, assists cardio-vascular disease, stomach cramps, gas, and intestinal spasms.

Lime assists apathy, anxiety, nervousness, depression, listlessness, refreshes a tired mind, is uplifting, stimulating, cheering, refreshing, makes a nice smelling deodorant, and is useful against alcoholism. **Caution:** Avoid direct sunlight exposure to the applied areas since it may be phototoxic. Descriptor: Anti-inflammatory, aids digestion, stimulates liver, antibiotic, alkalizing. Constituent: Aldehydes-Monoterpenes. Found in Peaceful Moments, Citrus Plus, and Serenity.

LIME, Organic Pressed Peel: USA (*Citrus aurantifolia*) – GRAS - Same as the Distilled Lime only it has a shorter shelf life. This is the Lime to use when taking internally. Descriptor: Stimulates liver, anti-inflammatory, aids digestion, alkalizing. Constituent: Monoterpenes/Aldehydes. Found in First Aid, Peacemaker, Faith, and Resp EZ.

LITSEA CUBEBA, Wild: China (*Litsea cubeba*) It is beneficial for depression, inflammation, infections, is an antiseptic, and an astringent. Litsea cubeba is beneficial for blemishes, acne, excessively oily skin and hair, fungal infections, dermatitis, insect repellant, respiratory tonic, asthma, bronco-dilator, assists high blood pressure and coronary heart disease, arteriosclerosis, and tumors. It may be diffused with pine or eucalyptus for cleaning a room. It assists in increasing milk flow for nursing mothers. It is very uplifting, stimulating, and useful for fatigue, lethargy, insomnia, anxiety and nervous depression. Descriptor: Anti-lipid stimulates liver, aids digestion, decongestant, anti-inflammatory. Constituent: Aldehydes/Sesquiterpenes. Found in Angel Assist and Peacemaker.

MANDARIN, Red: Italy Pressed Peel (*Citrus nobilis*) – GRAS - The French regarded it as a safe remedy for children and the elderly. It is beneficial for strengthening the liver, indigestion, hiccups, acne, congested and oily skin, scars, spots, stretch marks, toner, and fluid retention. It helps with PMS, menstrual cramps, obesity, dyspepsia, intestinal problems, detoxification, increases lymphatic circulation, and assists with insomnia caused by nervousness, nervous tension, and restlessness.

Aromatic influences: brings child-like energy and is a favorite of children. It signifies the inner child and assists in getting a 'handle' on routines. Descriptor: Alkalizing, aids digestion, tonic, stimulates liver, decongestant. Constituent: Esters/Monoterpenes. Found in Faith, Citrus Plus, Love, Spice Traders, Peacemaker, and In The Moment.

MARJORAM, Organically Grown: Egypt (*Origanum marjorana L.*) – GRAS – Assists the respiratory system, promotes intestinal peristalsis, and a digestive stimulant. Beneficial for infections, bacteria, spasms, tones the parasympathetic nervous system, for insomnia, nervous tension, lowering blood pressure, cramps, pain, menstrual problems, a sedative, and arterial vasodilator. It assists in draining blood from bruises and speeds the healing, migraine headaches, arthritis, muscular aches and stiffness, sprains, gas, sinusitis, chronic fatigue syndrome, and strains.

Marjoram assists with circulatory disorders, asthma, bronchitis, coughs, colic, colds, constipation, PMS, and dilates the blood vessels reducing the strain on the heart. Aromatic influences: peace and sleep. It may calm the emotions, provides comfort during times of grief, loneliness, and sadness. It is said to strengthen willpower. **Caution:** long-term use may permanently inhibit sex drive. Descriptor: Stimulates liver, aids digestion, antibiotic, decongestant.

Constituent: Monoterpenes. Found in Migraine Relief, Breathe EZ, Circle of Life, Relief, Nerve Repair, and Sport Pro.

MELALEUCA, Wild: Australia (*Melaleuca quinquinervera*) – GRAS – *Melaleuca quinquinervera* or True Niaouli as it is sometimes called is hard to find because it is often adulterated with other oils. It is a strong urinary, pulmonary, intestinal antiseptic fights infections, bacteria, fungus especially beneficial against Candida, tumors and assists rectal cancer, inflammation, parasites, viruses including "slow" viruses, and catarrh. It has hormone-like action on the hypothalamus, pituitary, adrenal axis, ovarian-testicular systems, assists male hormonal action, and impotence.

It helps viral hepatitis, slow digestion, ulcers, malaria, insect bites, rheumatoid arthritis, sinusitis, serious skin disease, acne, boils, and used before and after radiation treatments to give protection from deep radiation burns. It assists wrinkles, psoriasis, leprosy type ulcers, itchy, scaly skin, pus, cold abscesses, gangrenous wounds, scalp crusts, herpes, and shingles. It is beneficial as an adrenal stimulant, helps a sluggish liver, pancreas problems, and all respiratory complaints, helps colds, fevers, circulation, hemorrhoids, nausea, increases white blood cells, and antibody activity.

It is beneficial for scarlet fever, measles, mumps, smallpox, tetanus bacillus, swollen glands, and typhoid fever especially when diffused. When entering a sick room cover your face with a gauze mask impregnated with a few drops of Melaleuca or just spray around the room. Aromatic influences: clears head and assists concentration. Descriptor: Expectorant, anti-oxidant, stimulates liver, aids digestion, decongestant, antibiotic. Constituent: Oxides-Monoterpenes.

MELISSA, Organically Grown: France (*Melissa officinalis*) – GRAS – Another name for Melissa is Lemon Balm. In ancient times it was considered the best remedy for a troubled nervous system. It has a very soothing lemony smell that relieves tension, and is, with rose and neroli, one of the major essential oils of the heart energy center. It has powerful anti-viral constituents, is an anti-depressant, and anti-spasmodic beneficial for muscles spasm. It is used for nervousness, anxiety, calms circulation, lowers blood pressure, slows and strengthens the heart, eases palpitations due to crisis, unusual stimulation, excitement, or fear.

Melissa is beneficial for cold sores, herpes, shingles, helps stop bleeding wounds, insomnia, migraine, fatigue, neurasthenia, fungal infections, rapid breathing, asthma, bronchitis, chronic coughs, and colds with a headache. It is uplifting, dispels fear, emotional shock, grief, anger, helping deal with the past, bringing acceptance, and understanding. It is an insect repellant. Descriptor: Stimulates liver, aids digestion, decongestant, anti-inflammatory, anti-coagulant. Constituent: Mono/Sesquiterpenes-Courmarins. Found in Guardian and Uplifting.

MOUNTAIN SAVORY, Organically Grown: Hungary (Satureja montana) – It is effective against catarrh, fungus, viruses, spasms, major infections, has been used as a general tonic for the body, and an analgesic. It is an immune stimulant, eases arthritis, warms muscles, raises blood pressure, stimulates circulation, and assists hypotension. Effective against flu, colds, inflammation of lymph nodes, malaria, recurrent fevers, tuberculosis, digestive stimulant, regulates peristalsis, assists diarrhea, gas, constipation, nervous indigestion, and nervous fatigue. Mountain Savory has a high phenol content that makes it a strong antiseptic and assists with abscesses, burns, and cuts. It is known to assist the adrenal gland. Recent research suggests it may have anti-HIV activity. Constituent: Monoterpenes/Esters/Phenols. Descriptor: stimulates liver, decongestant, alkalizing, tonic, antibiotic, antiseptic.

MYRRH, Wild: Somalia-C02 extracted
(Commiphora myrrha) – GRAS – It fights fungus, inflammation, bacteria, viruses, infections, and is beneficial for hyper-thyroidism. It assists with diarrhea, dysentery, viral hepatitis, ulcers, bronchitis, asthma, expelling mucus, toning lungs, vaginal thrush, menstrual difficulties, recovery from illness, stretch marks, cleansing obstructions in the womb and relieving the itch and irritation of weeping eczema. Myrrh is beneficial for fungal infections such as athlete's foot, Candida, jock itch, and ringworm. It assists with chapped and cracked skin, mature complexion, wrinkles, sore throat, voice loss, gum infection, gingivitis, mouth ulcers, hemorrhoids, and boosts immunity by stimulating the production of white blood cells. It is toning to the digestive tract, reduces stomach gas, and acidity.

Myrrh is beneficial for fear, apathy, and feeling like you have no incentive, it balances upper and lower chakras, enhances visualization, brings up deep hidden emotions, and awakens awareness. It is soothing, calming, supporting, used to purify spiritual environments, overcoming irritability, emotional coldness, and connecting. Aromatic influences: spiritual awareness, uplifting, releases stuck emotions, and motivates one to move forward. Descriptor: Stimulates liver, aids digestion, decongestant, anti-inflammatory, anti-lipic. Constituent: Monoterpenes-Sesquiterpenes. Found in Balance, Exodus, Guardian, Joyful, DNA Repair, Toning, Meditation, Prosperity, and Vitality.

MYRTLE, Wild: Tunisia (Myrtus communis) – It is beneficial for respiratory problems, infections, and an immune stimulant. Because it is relative mild, it is very suitable to use for children's coughs and chest complaints. It is beneficial for smoker's cough, bronchitis, flu, colds, tuberculosis, sinus infection, uterine infection, and skin antiseptic. Myrtle is deodorizing and helps all pulmonary disorders. It assists hemorrhoids, varicose veins, Candida, diarrhea, liver, gall bladder stimulant, and sore throats (especially those caused by staph). It assists hormonal imbalance, is a prostate decongestant and hormone-like for regulating the ovaries. For hypothyroidism it increases activity and improves balance.
Myrtle is beneficial for wrinkles, psoriasis, scaling

skin, inflamed skin, acne, asthma, and a sedative for insomnia. It is neuro-balancing, soothes anger, fear, despair, fear of illness, death, lack of composure, distraction, and materialistic yearnings. Aromatic influences: to be open to love and beauty. Descriptor: Stimulates liver, decongestant, aids digestion, expectorant, antioxidant. Constituent: Monoterpenes/Oxides. Found in Breathe EZ, Purify, DNA Repair, and Vitality.

NARGARMOTHA, Wild: India *(Cyperus rotundus)* – It has a strong smell that you may have to get used to. It is beneficial as a stomachic and for removing parasites. It is helpful with bronco-pulmonary congestion, mucus, digestive upsets, scabies, and scanty periods. It may induce menstruation so avoid during pregnancy. Descriptor: Sedating, anti-lipic, antioxidant, antispasmodic, anti-inflammatory, expectorant. Constituent: Ketones/Sesquiterpenes-Oxides.

NEROLI, Organically Grown: Tunisia *(Citrus aurantium)* – It has been used by the Egyptians for healing the mind, body and spirit. It assists in brings everything into focus at the moment. Known to be beneficial for scars, stretch marks, thread veins, mature and sensitive skin, tones the complexion, wrinkles, palpitations, poor circulation, chronic diarrhea, colic, flatulence, spasm, and nervous dyspepsia. Neroli assists anxiety, depression, nervous tension, shock, stress related conditions, and emotional problems. Neroli comes from the blossoms of the bitter orange tree and Petitgrain Bigarade comes from the leaves. Constituent: Monoterpenes/Esters. Descriptor: Stimulates liver, aids digestion, decongestant, alkalizing, tonic. Found in Balance, In The Moment, Neroli Blend, Uplifting, Skin Care, and Hormone Balance.

NUTMEG, Organically Grown: Indonesia *(Myristica fragrans)* – GRAS – It has adrenal cortex-like activity supporting the adrenals and increasing energy. It is beneficial for fainting, nervous fatigue, strong psycho stimulant, invigorates, and activates the mind, may produce intense dreams in color. It decreases bad breath, assists intestinal infections,

frigidity, impotence, neuralgia the severe pain along the nerves, nervous fatigue, gout, muscle aches, and pains, rheumatism, arthritis, gas, poor circulation, heart stimulant, and chronic diarrhea.

Nutmeg assists digestion of starchy foods and fats and loss of appetite. It is known to ease sprains, strains, fatigue, and congestion after sports. Aromatic influence: adding zest, fun and enchantment to life. Descriptor: Stimulates liver, decongestant, aids digestion, antifungal. Constituent: Monoterpenes-Caprilic Acid. Found in Fortify, Spice Traders, Toning, Sport Pro, and Vitality.

ORANGE, Organic: USA Pressed Peel *(Citrus sinensis)* – GRAS – It assists nervous dyspepsia (impaired digestion), gingivitis, mouth ulcers, constipation, chronic diarrhea, very beneficial when used with Vitamin C since it enhances the absorption. Beneficial for bronchitis, flu, boosts immunity, lowers body temperature, cools a fever or warms chills. Orange assists lymphatic circulation, water retention, tonic, insomnia, reduces obesity, nervousness, cardiac spasm, palpitation, muscular spasm, inflammation, antiseptic, sedative, false angina, menopause, PMS, and brings joy to the heart. It balances the emotions either relaxing or stimulating as needed, inspiring harmony, awakening creativity, and promoting self-awareness.

Aromatic influences: joy, generosity, gratitude, and may prevent extreme seriousness. **Caution:** For some this may be a "hot" copal that may irritate the skin. Dilute with carrier oil. Constituent: Monoterpenes-Alcohols. Descriptor: Stimulates liver, aids digestion, decongestion, stimulant. Found in Gentle Healer, Hormone Balance, Creamsicle, Love, Meditation, Magnify, Joyful, Balance, Prosperity, Peaceful Moments, Calming, Citrus Plus, Rejuvenate, Serenity, Spice Traders, and Toning.

OREGANO, Wild: Turkey *(Origanum vulgare)* – GRAS – It is one of the strongest antibacterial oils and may be beneficial when a strong response to bacterial infection is needed. You can smell its power from the first moment the bottle is opened - the aroma is quite intense. It has a broad spectrum of bactericidal and anti-microbial action. It is beneficial against fungus, infections, parasites, viruses, is an antiseptic, immune-stimulant, balancing the metabolism, and strengthens the vital centers of the body. It is beneficial for chronic bronchitis, colds, whooping cough, pneumonia, asthma, chronic rheumatism, muscular pain, and pulmonary tuberculosis.

Use for warts, infected cuts, wounds, waterlogged skin, and facial tics. It is a tonic, stimulates the liver and spleen, sooths nervous stomach disorders, calms intestinal spasms, gas, laxative, and stimulates appetite. It is stimulating to the nerves, revives the senses (can ease deafness or painful noise in ears), migraines, mental disease, relieves imaginary diseases, and mental psychopathic conditions giving a feeling of well being.

When taken internally in olive oil add 1 to 2 drops first to the olive oil and then to warm water. It may be taken several times per day. It strengthens the immune system but use sparingly since it could be toxic to the liver, kidneys, and nerves. Studies on rats have shown oregano to be effective against lung tumors. **Caution:** Oregano is extremely "hot" and will irritate the skin so always dilute. A liver cleanse may be beneficial if using oregano often. Aromatic influences: strengthening and feeling self-secure. Descriptor: Aids digestion, stimulates liver, decongestant, alkalizing, tonic, antibiotic, antiseptic. Constituent: Monoterpenes/Esters/Phenols. Found in Fortify, Spice Traders, and Sport Pro.

PALMAROSA, Organically Grown: India
(*Cymbopogon martini*) – It is beneficial for skin problems, wrinkles, acne, Candida, rashes, scaly and flaky skin. It re-establishes the physiological balance by immediately calming and refreshing the skin. It is beneficial for sinusitis, thrush, sore throat, bronchitis, fights microbes, bacteria, viruses, infections, fungus, and is an antiseptic. It stimulants

digestion, circulation, is a muscle tonic, normalizes thyroid, nervous exhaustion, stress related conditions, morning fatigue, and irritability. It assists all types of healing. Aromatic influences: calming and uplifting. It clears the mind to assist with decision-making and helps to develop wisdom. When diffused it may speed the body's ability to heal. Constituent: Monoterpenes-Esters. Descriptor: Tonic, aids digestion, stimulates liver, decongestant, alkalizing. Found in Baby Soft.

PATCHOULI, Organically Grown: India
(*Pogostemon cablin*) – GRAS - It is an antiseptic beneficial for fungus infections such as athlete's foot, jock itch, and Candida. It assists with inflammation, fevers, nervous exhaustion, diarrhea, weight loss by curbing the appetite, toning and tightening the skin to prevent sagging after weight loss. Use for wrinkles, chapped skin, dandruff, skin allergies, impetigo, hives, eczema, acne, seborrhea, tissue regeneration, dermatitis, hemorrhoids, intestinal tract issues, lice, insect and snake bites, is an insecticide, and beneficial in controlling perspiration. Patchouli is grounding, strengthening and integrates energy to all areas of the body. Aromatic influences: diminish depression and eases anxiety. Assists in stress-related conditions, sharpening intellect, improving concentration, energy, and may increase money flow. Descriptor: anti-inflammatory, anti-lipic, alkalizing, anti-febrile. Constituent: Sesquiterpenes-Aldehydes. Found in Baby Soft, Dreamtime, Toning, Support, Prosperity, Serenity, Calming, and Peaceful Moments.

PENNYROYAL, Organically Grown: Turkey
(*Micromeria fruticosa L.*) – It is excellent oil for lung congestion, coughs, colds, bronchitis, and bronchial tract infections. Place one or two drops in a cup of hot water and inhale the vapors. It assists in reducing a fever by cooling the body, is a liver and spleen tonic, assist in sea sickness, intestinal colic, gout, female disorders, delayed menstruation and for painful menstrual cramps. Constituent: Ketones. Descriptor: sedative, anti-spasmodic, anti-coagulant. Found in Sport Pro.

PEPPERMINT: USA first distilled, India Organically Grown *(Mentha piperita)* – GRAS - Benefits the respiratory system, opens the sensory system, fights bacteria, inflammation, spasms, and is an antiseptic. It is stimulating and strengthening beneficial to use for shock, fatigue, nervous stress, reduces fevers, throat infections, headaches, migraines, and toothaches. Peppermint assists flu, colds, asthma, bronchitis, itchy skin, swelling, jet lag, arthritis, sinuses, motion sickness, nausea, chronic fatigue syndrome, vertigo, colic, acne, ringworm, heartburn, diarrhea, indigestion, halitosis, varicose veins, menstrual regularity, hot flashes, cramps, liver problems, dispels pride, and inferiority. It mixes well with all oils but should be used in small amounts.

For Poison Ivy it has been reported by adding peppermint to rubbing alcohol 10 to 50% peppermint and 90 to 50% alcohol it has taken away itching. Aromatic influences: purification, the conscious mind, energize, relieve mental fatigue, increases alertness, and improve concentration. (Peppermint – directly effects the brain's center, which triggers a sensation of fullness after a meal – Alan Hirsch, MD) Peppermint is good to add a little to shampoo. It deters lice & dandruff. It promotes hair growth as well as balances the pH levels on the head for healthy and shiny hair. Constituent: Monoterpenes-Ketones/Oxides. Descriptor: Stimulates liver, decongestant, aids digestion, expectorant, antioxidant. Found in Gentle Healer, Focus, Relief, Breathe EZ, Nerve Repair, Slim & Trim, Soothing Relief, True Blue, Freedom, Freedom Plus, Bug Free, Pain EZ, Meditation, Rejuvenate, DNA Repair, Sports Pro, Joyful, Migraine Relief, and Tummy Rub.

PETITGRAIN BIGARADE, Organically Grown: Paraguay *(Citrus aurantium var amara)* – This is the leaves from the Bitter Orange tree and Neroli comes from the blossoms. It is said to bring a positive energy and promote optimism. It is an immune stimulant, fights bacteria, infections, inflammation, and spasms. It is beneficial for acne, greasy skin and hair, boils and cellular, and tissue regeneration. Petitgrain eases breathing and nervous asthma, useful for all respiratory infections, relaxes nervous muscle spasms, useful for increasing muscle tone, eases joint pain, assists arterial circulation, eases palpitations, and cardiovascular spasms.

Petitgrain is beneficial for gas, insomnia, excessive perspiration, depression, nervous exhaustion, stress, mental fatigue, and gives mental clarity. It promotes a healthy self-esteem and trust in others, increases inner vision, stimulates the conscious mind, and clears perception. It is beneficial for panic, anger, anxiety, eases disharmony, and re-establishes nerve equilibrium. Constituent: Esters/Monoterpenes. Descriptor: Alkalizing, tonic, stimulates liver, assists digestion, decongestant. Found in Hormone Balance, Dreamtime, Toning, Circle of Life, and Utopia.

PINE, European Black, Wild: India (pinus nigra)- Beneficial for cuts, sores, arthritis, muscle aches, poor circulation, asthma, colds, flu, sore throats, urinary infections, stress, and nervous exhaustion.

PINE NEEDLES, Wild: Austria *(Pinus sylvestris)* – GRAS - The Scotch pine is one of the most useful and safest therapeutically to use. It was used by the Native Americans to prevent scurvy, repel lice, and fleas. Use for cuts, sores, excessive perspiration, scabies, arthritis, gout, muscular aches and pains, and poor circulation. Use for a sore throat, flu, colds, rheumatism, asthma, bronchitis, catarrh, coughs, sinusitis, cystitis, urinary infection, fatigue, nervous exhaustion, stress related conditions, and to balance the adrenal glands. Descriptor: Stimulates liver, aids digestion, decongestant, anti-inflammatory, anti-lipic. Constituent: Monoterpenes/Sesquiterpenes. Found in Breathe EZ, Meditation, Mountain Retreat, Toning, Resp EZ, and Joyful.

RAVINTSARA, Organic: Madagascar *(Cinnamomum camphora)* It is referred to as "the oil that heals" in Madagascar. This is another of the "universal oils" and may be used for many purposes. It fights infection, fungus, viruses, bacteria, is an anti-biotic, antiseptic, an expectorant, and supporting to the nerves. It assists respiratory problems, colds, bronchitis, sinusitis, sore throats, coughs, flu, lung infections, wounds, cuts, burns, liver, cholera, viral hepatitis, herpes, infectious mononucleosis, insomnia, muscle strain, and fatigue. Aromatic influences: assists with realizing one's potential, self- esteem, increases desire for change, nervous fatigue, and relieves depression. Descriptor: Aids digestion, decongestant, expectorant, antioxidant. Constituent: Monoterpenes/Oxides. Found in Breathe EZ. Hair Support, and Rejuvenate.

ROSE, Organic: Bulgaria *(Rosa damascena)* – GRAS – It has an extraordinarily complex chemistry with over 300 known constituents. Rose enhances the frequency of every cell, bringing balance, and harmony to the body making it excellent for babies. It is said to fight depression, infections, spasms, bacteria especially diphtheria, strep, staph, E. coli, and anthrax. It is an immune stimulant, antiseptic a diuretic, tonic for the heart and liver, nerve sedative, inflamed gallbladder, laxative, stomachic, nausea, diarrhea, vomiting, assists gastro-intestinal ulcers, regulates the appetite, mouth ulcers, thrush, and gingivitis.

It is beneficial for chronic and bronchial asthma, bronchitis, tuberculosis, hay fever, sore throats, sedative for contusions and sprains, poor circulation, lowers high blood pressure, palpitations, arrhythmia, hemorrhaging, and lowers cholesterol. Rose assists to prevent scarring, skin disease, heal wounds, wrinkles, broken capillaries, eczema, herpes, conjunctivitis, shingles, radiation burns, ulcers, revitalizes, and rejuvenates dry, sensitive, and aging skin. It is beneficial for hangovers, diphtheria, urinary infections, assists irregular menstruation, and period pain.

Rose assists psychological impotence, frigidity, sterility, and sexual weakness in males and females when taken along with Vitamin A. Aromatic influences: creates a sense of well being, stimulating and elevating to the mind, helps release past hurts, and brings a feeling of love. Constituent: Monoterpenes/Sesquiterpenes-Oxides. Descriptor:

Stimulates liver, aids digestion, decongestant, anti-lipic, anti-inflammatory, expectorant, antioxidant Found in Baby Soft, Balance, Faith, Grateful, Love, In The Moment, Guardian, Magnify, Rose Blend, DNA Repair, Skin Care, and Utopia.

ROSEMARY, Organically Grown: Hungary *(Rosmarinus officinalis)* – GRAS - A general all around oil and another of the "Universal Oils". It is beneficial as a restorative, against spasms, viruses, bacteria, infections, and catarrh (clears mucus quickly), bronchitis, asthma, whooping cough, colds, and flu. It assists the immune and endocrine systems, regulates ovaries and testicular functions, mental fatigue, Candida, sinusitis, viral hepatitis, diabetes, cholera, disorientation, excellent for morning stimulation and energy, clears and awakens the brain, lethargy, assists speech, hearing, sight, and assists in opening the throat chakra. It is beneficial for headaches, migraines, dandruff, lice, strengthens and promotes hair growth, cellulite, fluid retention, and irregular periods.

Rosemary regenerates and builds connective tissue, lowers blood pressure and blood cholesterol. It assists skin infections, poor circulation, promotes new cell growth, seborrhea, angina, varicose veins, gout, arthritis, colitis, rheumatism, anemia, jaundice, stress, nervous and physical exhaustion, muscular spasms, and sprains. Benefits kidney and liver problems, stimulates liver metabolism and gall bladder action (bile), assists enlarged liver-cirrhosis and protects liver cells, analgesic, strengthens the body, and controls mood swings.

Aromatic influences: longevity, clear thought, memory, conscious mind, uplifting, and love. Arouses ambition and drive, inspires the desire to achieve, and strengthens willpower. Descriptor: Stimulates liver, aids digestion, decongestant, sedative, antispasmodic, analgesic. Constituent: Monoterpenes/Ketones. Found in Gentle Healer, DNA Repair, Focus, Fortify, Hair Support, Purify, Spice Traders, and Resp EZ.

ROSEWOOD, Wild: Brazil (*Aniba roseodora*) – It fights infections, bacteria, viruses, fungus, parasites, and is an antiseptic. It is a cell stimulant and tissue regenerator creating skin elasticity, soothing skin problems, (balancing skin, clearing blemishes and improving acne) and slows aging. It is beneficial for Candida, scars, wounds, colds, ticklish coughs, sore throats, fevers, immune stimulant, and for all bronco-pulmonary infections especially in babies.

It assists with frigidity, nervous tension, stress, depression, relieves nausea with headaches, stabilizes and balances the Central Nervous System. It is an overall tonic relaxant, asthenia, low energy, overwork, jet lag, promotes alertness and assists suffers of sexual abuse. Aromatic influences: peace, gentleness, calming, and relaxing the nerves. It helps to relieve anxiety, stress, balances emotions, and kills airborne bacteria. Descriptor: Stimulates liver, aids digestion, decongestant, anti-oxidant, expectorant. Constituent: Monoterpenes-Oxides. Found in Baby Soft, Balance, Confidence, and Guardian.

SAGE, Wild: Turkey (*Salvia fruticosa miller*) – GRAS - The wild sage is milder than the cultivated sage making it beneficial for children. It is used for strengthening the vital center, skin conditions, acne, eczema, dandruff, and hair loss. Sage may assist metabolism, menopause, is a general stimulant, activating the nervous system and adrenal cortex. It is a diuretic, antiseptic, anti-cancer, anti-spasmodic, beneficial for the lymphatic, digestion, liver, urinary and pulmonary systems. It is known to help with chronic bronchitis, asthma, night sweats, glandular disorders by improving the estrogen, progesterone and testosterone balance, assists menstrual irregularity, gingivitis, bacterial infections, sprains, catarrh, arthritis, rheumatism, is a disinfectant, and astringent. Aromatic influences: relieving strain, depression, and mental fatigue. Constituent: Oxides/Ketones. Descriptor: Expectorant, sedative, antioxidant, antispasmodic, analgesic. Found in Hair Support, Balance, Vitality, and Support.

SANDALWOOD, Wild: India (Santalum *album*) – GRAS – It is beneficial for depression, nerve sedative, urinary and pulmonary problems, an antiseptic, astringent, and stimulates the immune system. It fights infections, bacteria, fungus, spasms, and decongests the lymph system. It assists and balances any skin type or condition (dry, aged, cracked, chapped, psoriasis, and eczema), increases water retention of collagen, increases capillary circulation, the connective tissue, and dermis are strengthened and moisturized.

Sandalwood is wonderful for the hair and scalp. It assists cardiac fatigue, sciatica, muscle spasms, hemorrhoids, neuralgia, and any inflammation or congestion of the kidneys and bladder. It is used for bronchitis, dry persistent coughs, catarrh, sinusitis, sore throat, strep, staph, nausea, earaches, laryngitis, cholera, diarrhea, gastritis, cystitis, urinary, aphrodisiac, impotence, gonorrhea, pelvic and prostate congestion, and menstrual problems. It increases fat metabolism, aids digestion, insomnia, and is a heart tonic.

It assists with stress, past ties, grief, obsessions, feelings of isolation and aggression, and egocentric behavior. It assists in removing negative programming from the cells, increases oxygen around the pituitary and pineal glands, and is found to be supportive in cases of fear and low self-confidence. Aromatic influences: meditation, quieting, and healing. Descriptor: Antispasmodic, anti-inflammatory, sedative, anti-febrile. Constituent: Sesquiterpenes-Aldehydes/Ketones. Found in Peacemaker, DNA Repair, Sandalwoods, Utopia, Hormone Balance, Break Thru, In The Moment, Guardian, Dreamtime, Peacemaker, Balance, Peaceful Moments, and Rejuvenate.

SPEARMINT, Organically grown: India (*Mentha spicata*) – GRAS – It benefits all respiratory problems, refreshing to the muscles, nervous, and glandular systems. It assists in balancing the metabolism, is antiseptic, beneficial against fungus, infections, parasites, inflammation, and spasms. It is helpful for bronchitis, catarrh, bad breath, sore gums, hiccups, hypertension, Candida, flatulence, indigestion, intestinal cramps, eases labor, and reduces milk.

Spearmint is beneficial for flu, fevers, colic, releases retention of urine, nausea, fatigue, headache, migraine, neurasthenia stress (exhaustion), and nervous strain. It is hormone-like in that it may release emotional blocks and bring balance. It brings child-like innocence and lightness. Aromatic influences: peace, happiness, and clarity. Descriptor: Antispasmodic, sedative, antispasmodic, decongestant, stimulates liver, aids digestion, expectorant, antioxidant. Constituent: Ketones/Monoterpenes/ Oxides. Found in Vitality, Gentle Healer, and Rejuvenate.

SPIKENARD, Wild: Nepal (*Nardostachys jatamansi*) – It is sometimes called Jatamansi. It is one of the most effective oils for supporting a calm mind and balanced nervous system. Highly revered for its ability to support deep sleep, help one work with and release subconscious trauma. It is good to use for grief after losing a loved one. It is beneficial for Candida, incurable skin problems, regenerates all functions and layers of the skin, wound healing, inflammation, menstrual difficulties, regulates hormonal system when imbalanced, and stimulates the ovaries. Spikenard balances Sympathetic with Parasympathetic functions, calms restlessness, intensifies feelings toward a spiritual teacher, inspires devotion, generosity, and deep inner peace. It is mentioned in the Bible. Constituent: Esters-Monoterpenes. Descriptor: Sedative, alkalizing, expectorant. Found in Exodus, Meditation, and Support.

SPRUCE, Wild: Canada (*Tsuga canadensis*) – GRAS – It fights infection, inflammation, microbes, spasms, is an astringent, expectorant, general tonic and antiseptic. It supports the respiratory, nervous, and glandular systems, is a diuretic, diaphoretic and strengthens the immune system. Spruce is mentally grounding, restores depleted adrenal glands,

balances the solar plexus, stimulates the thymus, and has cortisone-like properties.

Spruce is beneficial for Candida, bone pain, rheumatism, arthritis, joints, sciatica, poor circulation, hyper-thyroidism, colds, flu, prostate, anxiety, and stress. Aromatic influences: elevating and opening to bring about a balance of emotions. Descriptor: Stimulates liver, aids digestion, anti-lipic, decongestant, anti-inflammatory, alkalizing, tonic. Constituent: Monoterpenes-Sesquiterpenes-Esters. Found in Breathe EZ, Confidence, Guardian, Joyful, Meditation, Mountain Retreat, Prosperity, Balance, Soothing Relief, True Blue, Utopia, and Toning.

TAGETES, Organically Grown: Zimbabwe (*Tagetes erecta*) – It fights infections, inflammation, microbes, spasms, fungus, and parasites especially roundworms. It is a stomachic, effective for digestive system and helps Candida infection. It is a sedative, beneficial for slow healing wounds, burns, cuts, bruises, catarrh, and respiratory infections, dilates bronchi, eases mucus, congestion, coughs, aches, pains, strains, and lowers blood pressure. Aromatic influences: clears thinking, relieves tension, and assists emotional control. Descriptor: Sedative, calming, antispasmodic, stimulates liver, aids digestion, decongestant Constituent: Ketones-Monoterpenes. Tagetes has its own distinct smell that can be quite offensive for some people.

TANGERINE: USA Pressed Peel: (*Citrus reticulata*) – GRAS – It supports and strengthens the lymphatic, digestive and nervous systems. A chemical found in tangerine is very effective in shrinking tumors when applied over the area. It reduces excess fluid, obesity, smoothes out stretch marks, helps break down cellulite fat pockets, diarrhea, laxative, inflammation, cramps, parasites, intestinal spasm, muscle spasms, constipation, tired aching limbs, circulation in the extremities, and calms the nerves. Tangerine stimulates the liver and gall bladder, gas, belching, cramps, PMS, dizziness, anxiety, hypnotic effect, stress, tension, and soothing. Aromatic influences: relieving emotional grief and stress, fear, cheering, inspires, assisting to bring about a sense of peace. Descriptor: Stimulates liver, aids digestion, calming, decongestant, alkalizing, anti-febrile. Constituent: Monoterpenes-Aldehydes. Found in Serenity, Citrus Plus, Passion for Life, Calming, and Peacemaker.

TARRAGON, Organically Grown: Yugoslavia (*Artemisia dracunculus*) – GRAS – It assists inflammation, anti-cancerous, neuromuscular spasms, infections, parasites, viruses and bacteria. Tarragon assists and balances intestinal activity relieving discomfort, upset stomach from emotional distress, relieves any kind of colitis (inflammatory and spasmodic), dyspepsia, gas, nervous and sluggish digestion, and prevents fermentation. It is beneficial for sciatica, urinary tract infection, pre-menstrual discomfort and pain, hiccups, gout, arthritis, rheumatic, heart spasms, palpitations, and is a general circulatory stimulant. Tarragon is an immune strengthener, reduces physical weakness, nausea, anorexia, intestinal spasm, and eases abnormal tendency for convulsions. Aromatic influences: allows one to digest and assimilate new ideas. Descriptor: Alkalizing, antispasmodic, anti-febrile, adaptogenic, calming. Constituent: Phenolpropanes-Aldehydes/Courmarins Found in Tummy Rub.

TEA TREE, Wild: Australia (*Melaleuca alternifolia*) – It is beneficial against inflammation, viruses, fungus, bacteria, parasites, infections (especially against staph, strap, respiratory, ear, nose and throat infections) and against such infectious diseases as chickenpox. Tea Tree heals wounds, fungal infections, athlete's foot, Candida, jock itch, gum disease, rashes, lice, sunburn, digestion, diarrhea, vaginal thrush, and abscess. It is beneficial for acne, cold sores, herpes, burns, shock, hysteria, warts, colds, flu, tuberculosis, sinusitis, whooping cough, tissue regenerator, stimulates lymphatic circulation, and is an immune stimulant. Tea Tree is an antiseptic and insecticide. Aromatic influences: cleansing, energy stimulant, and nervous depression. Descriptor: Stimulates liver, aids digestion, decongestant, anti-lipic, anti-

inflammatory, expectorant, antioxidant. Constituent: Monoterpenes/Sesquiterpenes/ Oxides. Found in Gentle Healer and Purify.

THYME, Organically Grown: Hungary (*Thymus vulgaris*) – GRAS – It is beneficial against microbes, bacteria, fungus, infections, viruses, inflammation, parasites, and is an antiseptic. It works as a neuro and cardio-tonic builds the immune system by stimulating the white blood cells into action, assists in overcoming emotional fatigue, and physical weakness especially after an illness. It is very strengthening to the nerves, assists memory, feeling depressed, colitis, sinusitis, congestion, dyspepsia, general tonic for stomach, diarrhea, chills, infectious colitis, and poor circulation. Thyme is beneficial for bronchitis, asthma, tonsillitis, whooping cough, cystitis, tuberculosis, urinary, anthrax, warts, abscess, sciatica, lumbago, bruises, burns, insect bites, lice, raises low blood pressure, sprains, sporting injuries, headache, and insomnia.

To protect your lungs during a cold or flu, make a chest rub with one teaspoon olive oil and 3-4 drops of thyme oil. The warming vapors will keep your respiratory passages open and moist even as they fight infections with their antiseptic action. For dandruff control dilute four drops of thyme oil in one teaspoon olive oil and apply on the scalp one hour before washing your hair. Then, after shampooing, rinse your hair with six drops of thyme added to one quart of water. Aromatic influences: Assist in supplying energy in times of physical weakness and stress, releases mental blocks, calms and relaxes anger, frustration, and gives courage. Descriptor: Stimulates liver, expectorant, antioxidant, aids digestion, decongestant. Constituent: Oxides-Monoterpenes. Found in Bug Free, Spice Traders, and Sport Pro.

VALERIAN ROOT, Wild: Himalaya (*Valeriana jatamansi*) – GRAS – It has been highly esteemed since medieval times and was called "all heal." Valerian sedates the nervous system and helps put a damper on the pain of shingles, a virus that affects the nerves and usually appears when under stress. Massage a few drops around the area. It assists digestion, stimulates the liver, and is excellent for insomnia, nervous indigestion, muscle spasms, heart pain, palpitations, neuralgia, fevers, intestinal colic, rheumatism, restlessness, tension, agitation, panic attacks, and as a pain reliever for migraines. Descriptor: Stimulates liver, aids digestion, tonic, decongestant, alkalizing, sedative. Constituent: Monoterpenes-Sesquiterpenes/Esters. Found in Utopia.

VANILLA, Organically Grown: Madagascar *(Vanilla planifolia)* – GRAS - Beneficial as a nerve sedative, induces menstruation, calms emotions, eases tensions, anger, frustration, and brings warm memories. Constituent: Aldehyde. Descriptor: Sedative, calming. Found in Citrus Plus, In The Moment, Creamsicle, and Vanilla Blend.

VETIVER, Wild: Haiti, Hydro-distilled *(Vetivera zizanioides)* – It is beneficial for acne, cuts, oily skin, dry mature aging skin, softens, hydrates, detoxifies connective tissue and epidermis through capillary simulation, cell regenerator, and eases masculine aging signs. It assists arthritis, muscular aches and pains, rheumatism, sprains, stiffness, stimulates circulation, fortifies red blood cells, lymph, increases oxygen, and assists a depressed immune system.

It is a tonic to the urinary system, stimulates the cells' restorative power, assists impotence, pancreas stimulant, and assists liver congestion. It eases post-partum depression, insomnia, mental and physical exhaustion balances the Central Nervous System, and helps in easing off tranquilizers. Aromatic influences: grounding and stimulates for more vitality, cleans and strengthens the aura. It is deeply relaxing and very valuable for massage and in the bath for anyone experiencing stress. Constituent: Sesquiterpenes-Monoterpenes. Descriptor: Sedative, anti-inflammatory, stimulates liver and pancreas. Found in Passion for Life, Toning, Hormone Balance, Grounding, and Soothing Relief.

VITEX BERRY, Wild: Isle of Crete (Vitex agnus castus) – Traditionally used for female hormonal problems, helping to resume halted menstrual bleeding, stopping cramps, depression, relieving breast pains, and swelling. It relaxes the nerves, frees spasms, relieves pain, calms the liver, regulates the pituitary, and harmonizes the endocrine system. It is known for its benefits as a tonic, decongestant, stimulant and relaxant action on liver, intestines, and uterus. Vitex Berry has been found to be 89% successful in remission of Parkinson's disease in laboratory animals. It may be beneficial used in the Rejuvenation Technique on the ankles or the feet. **Caution:** Should not be used during pregnancy since it is a uterine stimulant. Descriptor: Aids digestion, uterine stimulant, tonic, stimulates liver. Constituent: Monoterpenes.

WINTERGREEN, Organic: Nepal *(Gaultheria fragrantissima)* – It is beneficial for muscle and joint discomfort, arthritis, cellulite, obesity, poor circulation, edema, and headaches from liver congestion. It stimulates the liver, beneficial for heart disease, hypertension, rheumatism, is anti-inflammatory, tendentious, cramps, and high in cortisone-like functions. It is beneficial for eczema, hair care, psoriasis, gout, ulcers, broken or bruised bones. Avoid prolong exposure to this oil due to toxic build up in the liver. Descriptor: Alkalizing, antispasmodic. Constituent: Esters. Found in Soothing Relief and True Blue.

YARROW, BLUE, Organically Grown: Hungary *(Achillea millefolium)* An age-old herbal medicine used for complaints including fever, respiratory infections, digestive problems, sores, severe rashes, wounds, and nervous conditions. It is very beneficial for the skin, scalp, and known to promote hair growth. It assists inflammation, aids digestion, and is a sedative. Constituent: Monoterpenes-Ketones. Descriptor: Inflammation, aids digestion, sedative.

YLANG YLANG COMPLETE, Organically Grown: Comores and YLANG YLANG EXTRA, Organic: Madagascar *(Cananga odorata genuina)* – GRAS - The Ylang Ylang Extra, the first extraction, is more concentrated, and may achieve faster results. It is calming, relaxing, and soothing to nervous system. It also assists with anxiety, depression, and poor self esteem. It helps in balancing the equilibrium, heart function, is a general tonic, anti-spasmodic, assists high blood pressure, palpitations, tachycardia, arterial hypertension, mental fatigue, insomnia, and lowers abnormally fast breathing.

Ylang Ylang is beneficial for diabetes, hair loss, wrinkles, and balancing oily skin. Aromatic influences: dispelling anger, emotional coldness, tension, frustration, balancing, love and enhancing relationships. Descriptor: Sedative, Aphrodisiac, nerves. Constituent: Esters/Phenols-Sesquiterpenes. Found in Calming, Peaceful Moments, Baby Soft, Break Thru, Circle of Life, Love, Faith, Grateful, Guardian, Hair Support, Magnify, Mountain Retreat, Peacemaker, Balance, DNA Repair, Serenity, and Uplifting.

It is good to know the difference between synergies and blends as they are used in this book. When complimentary pure essential oils are mixed together, they are called a synergy. The benefit of the synergy oils is much greater than using the same single oil separately. When carrier oil such as fractionated coconut oil is mixed with the synergy they are then called blends.

In this section it is explained why a synergy or blend was formulated and the oils that were used in the formulation. Since all the benefits of each oil are not listed, it will be helpful for you to go back to the Singles Section and read about each oil in that synergy or blend to understand more of their benefits.

Applying essential oils to the bottom of the feet is always a good way to start using them. The "application" comments in the following text discuss other applications that may be used. Information on the Vita Flex Technique is explained later in this book.

My favorite way to use the oils is on the bottom of my feet morning and night. Each morning I think of what I want to accomplish during the day and apply one or more oils. Focus, Magnify, or Mountain Retreat help keep me focused on moving towards my goals and avoiding judging others. If I am going to be out among a lot of people, I will use Fortify or Defense for protection from sickness and disease. And when I go shopping I always use Prosperity on my feet and wrists to ensure finding the items I am looking for at a good price.

Confidence gives me the courage to be myself when I am sharing with others. Before bed I like to use Dreamtime or Serenity on my feet or Love over my heart. The essential oils are so delightful! There are many different combinations you can use to match, change or enhance your moods. Enjoy the excitement of using oils.

Please remember the following when working with essential oils: Keep out of the reach of children. Avoid contact with eyes. Avoid dropping the pure oils in the ears. Generally, it is best to rub the oils on the skin but there are times when taking them internally is beneficial. Always dilute "hot" oils with carrier oil or something with a fat content like cream.

~~~~~~~~~

ANGEL ASSIST:
Contains – Geranium, Cypress, Litsea Cubeba, Clary Sage, and Black Pepper
It was formulated to be used in times of personal challenges and change when extra assistance is desired. It assists in the transition of life's course, in letting go of the negative past, and when there is fear of the future. It eases the anxiety and tension of mentally and physically demanding days, helps in overcoming fear, and of expressing oneself in a positive, loving way.

Angel Assist motivates one into action and gives the courage to move forward. It helps in eliminating blocked personal growth, indecision, emotional wounds, is stabilizing, and brings peace. It assists in healing the heart and bringing out the inner child. Aromatic Influence: grounding, very calming, increased spiritual awareness, and self-control. It helps in calling in the Angelic Force to assist you.

Traditional Application: across the forehead, on the ears, temples, wrists, throat, and over the heart. This oil is great in a massage. **Companion Oils:** Love, Peacemaker, Rose, and Grateful.

BABY SOFT:
Contains - Rosewood, Palmarosa, Elemi, Ylang Ylang Extra, Geranium, Patchouli, and Rose
Beneficial for general skin care, assists with dermatitis, acne, broken capillaries, oily skin, rashes, and congested, mature, scaly or flaky skin. The oils in this blend benefit skin regeneration, scarring, are used to prevent and retard wrinkles, enhance youthful appearance, and assist skin

elasticity. Baby Soft is calming, assists in slowing the aging process, very soothing for skin problems and wound healing, especially after facial surgery. It is beneficial against microbes, bacteria, viruses, fungus, infections, and re-establishes the balance of the skin.

It is exceptional when used for a baby oil to avoid possible harmful effects of the mineral oil in commercial baby oils. It is important to dilute before using on the baby by putting one drop in ten drops of carrier oil. Baby Soft has been used with excellent results for diaper rash and teenage skin. Men may use it for chapped skin or as an after-shave. It may relieve stress during pregnancy and be of benefit during the birthing process.

Traditional Application: applied to inner ankles, across lower back, and abdomen during pregnancy. Approximately two weeks prior to delivery massage perineum daily. This may assist in avoiding an episiotomy by preparing the body to stretch. Baby Soft is excellent diluted with massage oil for a full body massage, wear as a perfume, night cream, and added to bath water. When using as baby oil add three to five drops to 1/4 oz massage oil. For teenage skin, put ten drops of Baby Soft in a 4 oz-spray bottle. Fill bottle with water that has been boiled and cooled or use bottled water. Shake before using and spritz face several times during the day. It works well when sprayed on sunburns. **Companion Oils:** Frankincense, Myrrh, Elemi, Sandalwood, Neroli, Spikenard, and Skin Care.

BALANCE:
Contains - Hyssop, Lavender, Lemon, Orange, Geranium, Rosewood, Sandalwood, Myrrh, Sage, Spruce, Frankincense, Rose Otto, German Chamomile, Ylang Ylang Extra, Neroli, and Angelica root
It unlocks the energy centers allowing energy to flow more efficiently through the body promoting balance and emotional healing. We need to be in harmony with ourselves, our creator, and the world around us before we may truly feel and overcome our negative emotions. It is beneficial in reducing stress and generating a feeling of well-being, relaxation, and peace as it unblocks the energy centers.

Traditional Application: apply to each of the energy centers, on the ears, over the heart, and over the areas of poor circulation. When there is an allergy or irritation to the smell of an essential oil, place one drop of Balance on the tips of your fingers and massage the center of the forehead clockwise (clockwise means to pretend the face of the clock in on your body and rotate your hand just as the hands on the clock would go) for about 30 seconds. Then massage the thymus, at the base of the throat, in a clockwise motion for 30 seconds. (Pretend the face of the clock in on the forehead and thymus.) This will assist in bring balance. It may help addictions when rubbed on the jaw several times a day.

Because this blend contains ten oils that are very beneficial and specific for skin problems it is good for all skin conditions. Put 15 drops in ½ oz of Jojoba or FCO and use on the body after a bath or apply as a night cream to the face. This will also assist in releasing and balancing negative emotions during sleep. **Companion Oils:** Rose, Neroli, Love, Uplifting, Grateful, and Magnify.

BRAIN POWER:
Contains - Ylang Ylang Extra, Melissa, Sandalwood, Frankincense, Cedarwood, Lavender, and Helichrysum italicum
It assists the brain when extra thinking power is needed or when there has been an injury to the head. High in sesquiterpenes these oils cross the blood brain barrier and assists in carrying oxygen to the pineal and pituitary glands. It helps to develop greater focus, clear mental cobwebs and is beneficial when used for meditation. It produces a calming, uplifting, soothing, elevated mental state bringing peace. It acts as a sedative to overcome anger and stress related conditions. It assists in overcoming grief, anxiety, depression, fear, mental fatigue, and poor self-esteem.

The military conducted an experiment in which DNA was placed in a container from which they could measure changes in the DNA. Twenty-eight vials of DNA were given (one each) to 28 researchers trained in how to generate and feel feelings and each had strong emotions. It was discovered that the DNA changed its shape according to the feelings of the researchers. When the researchers felt appreciation, gratitude, and love, the DNA responded by relaxing, the strands unwound, and the length of the DNA became longer. When the researchers felt anger, fear, stress, or frustration, the DNA responded by tightening up, becoming shorter and switched off many of the DNA codes.

If you've ever felt "shut down" by negative emotions, now you know why your body was equally shut down too. The researchers found that the shutdown DNA codes could be reversed and turned back on again when feelings of love, gratitude, appreciation, and joy were felt by them. Brain Power creates this balancing effect assisting the DNA codes to relax, soothing the nervous system, balancing the equilibrium, and heart function. When we get angry or won't forgive we create barriers that keep us from going forward. It assists in balancing extremes in emotions, bringing peace, personal growth, and joy back into our life.

Traditional Application: Apply on the back of the neck, on the temples, the bottoms of the feet, and especially on the big toe massaging for several minutes. **Companion Oils:** Rosemary, Basil, Peppermint, Helichrysum, Nerve Repair, and Focus.

BREAK THRU:
Contains - Lavender, Rose Geranium, Elemi, Sandalwood, Blue Tansy, Ylang Ylang Extra, German Chamomile, and Cypress
It was formulated with the objective of enhancing the release of memory trauma from both the cells of the liver, which stores anger and hate emotions, and the trauma center in the brain. These oils assists in letting go of negative emotions and frustration easily and gently with love and forgiveness. It assists in moving emotions in a more effective and efficient way. We still remember the experience, but the pain is gone. It has been reported to be a support when working on breaking free from addictions.

Traditional Application: massage a few drops of Break Thru on the liver and then apply a hot wet towel compress over the liver. Put a drop on the temples and on the ears. Place a drop on your hands, rub your hands together, cup them over your nose, and inhale. **Companion Oils:** Grateful, Angel Assist, Balance, Utopia, Serenity, Mountain Retreat, and Guardian.

Comments: Always begin by cleansing the colon before detoxifying the liver. Ten days after starting the colon cleanse add the liver cleanse. After you have been on the liver cleanse at least a week do the following: 1st- put Calming on the bottom of the feet, 2nd- put Balance on energy centers, and 3rd- alternate using Tummy Rub and Break Thru over the liver with a hot compress for several days.

BREATHE EZ:
Contains - Eucalyptus globulus, Eucalyptus citriodora, Myrtle, Eucalyptus radiata, Peppermint, Spruce, Ravintsara, Pine, and Marjoram
It was formulated to assist the respiratory system and be beneficial for bronchitis, pneumonia, flu, colds, fevers, asthma, laryngitis, coughs, sinusitis, sore throats, cold sores, and lung infections. It loosens and expels mucus and reduces inflammation. It is beneficial for anything viral, bacterial, fungal, and infections.

It supports the nerves, calms the emotions, and comforts young children. It assists the regeneration of lung tissue, is beneficial for infections, and skin diseases such as chicken pox. It is beneficial for spasms, cramps, swelling, muscle aches and stiffness, nervous mental exhaustion and stress related conditions. It assists digestion, stimulates the thymus, boosts energy, and is an immune booster.

Breathe EZ has been known to assist in getting rid of bone spurs, in listening to our spirit, having the courage to speak our truth honestly, openly, effectively, and appropriately. It removes the traumas that keep us from breathing in and experiencing the fullness of life.

Traditional Application: massage topically to the lungs and throat areas. Apply a hot, wet towel compress for 15 minutes. Beneficial for respiratory conditions by putting a few drops on the pillowcase or used in a suppository application with massage oil. Another application is to mix 20 drops of Breathe EZ with 10 drops of Frankincense in ½ oz of carrier oil. Put mixture into a syringe and implant into the rectum at night. Retain the solution all night, when it is in carrier oil it takes longer to be absorbed. Repeat each night for up to ten nights in a row and if not better, rest for four days and repeat again for ten more days. For children use one-half to one-third the amount.

Diffusing Breathe EZ has been a powerful treatment for viral TB, pneumonia, and other viral problems. Apply to Vita Flex points on the feet. **Caution:** Asthmatics may react to Eucalyptus globulus. Use with caution. **Companion Oils:** Fortify, Exodus, Spice Traders, Cypress, Rosemary, and Resp EZ.

BUG FREE:
Contains – Citronella, Cedarwood, Lavender, Peppermint, Eucalyptus, Thyme and Lemongrass
Bug Free was formulated to assist with detouring mosquitoes, flees, ticks, lice, and other insects.
Traditional Application: Apply to exposed skin before going out. **Companion Oils:** Add more drops of Cedarwood to prevent bedbugs, Buzz Off Spray, Eucalyptus, and Citronella.

CALMING:
Contains – Tangerine, Ylang Ylang Complete, Orange, Blue Tansy, and Patchouli
Calming is composed of oils known for their calming effects. It creates a sense of well-being and promotes relaxation. Beneficial for insomnia, worries, it is very soothing, brings patience, inspires harmony, joy, gratitude, and balances emotions. This is a wonderful oil to diffuse. It calms tensions

and stress, diminishes depression, eases anxiety, and is uplifting giving a sense of deep peace.

Traditional Application: massaging on the bottom of feet before bed may assist in a peaceful nights rest. Calming is especially beneficial for children after an overactive or stressful day. **Companion Oils:** Creamsicle, Serenity, and Peaceful Moments.

CINNAMON BLEND:
Contains – Cinnamon and FCO
Cinnamon Bark by itself is very hot and will burn the skin. Here it is blended with FCO and in most cases is safe to use right from the bottle (for sensitive skin do a skin test first). It assists circulation, lowering glucose, strengthening the heart, endocrine and nervous systems. It is an immune stimulant working against infections, bacteria, fungus, viruses, and parasites. It is used against typhoid, tropical infection, flu, colds, coughs, rheumatism, and warts. It is a general all around maintenance oil. It is a powerful purifier and enhances the action and activity of the other oils. Aromatic influences: May promote physical energy, psychic awareness, and increasing one's prosperity.

Traditional Application: Cinnamon Blend is beneficial applied to the feet. It is also good to use in cooking and herb teas. **Companion Oils:** Fortify, Freedom Plus, Spice Traders, Thyme, Oregano, Black Cumin, and Ravintsara.

CIRCLE OF LIFE:
Contains - Cypress, Marjoram, Hyssop, Eucalyptus citriodora, Ylang Ylang Extra, Helichrysum italicum, Ginger Root, and Petitgrain Combava
This formulation assists in strengthening and improving cardiovascular function. It gives energy, improves circulation, tightens tissues and balances the equilibrium, heart functions and palpitations. It is effective against bacteria, viruses, opening the respiratory system, assists swollen glands, nervous exhaustion and anxiety, dispels anger and assists in healing emotions, creating a feeling of security, and grounding.

Circle of Life promotes health and assists in recuperating from long illnesses. It is soothing, calming, balancing, providing comfort during times of grief, loneliness, sadness, and uncontrolled crying or talking. It is very uplifting, comforting, gives courage, peace, assists in visualization, self-esteem, and personal growth. It may also assist in lowering blood pressure, reducing stress, and alleviating hemorrhoids.

Traditional Application: massage the chest area and heart, on the left hand below the ring finger, the Vita Flex point on the left arm just above the elbow, on the toes and along the spine from C4 to T5. For varicose veins add a few drops each of Circle of Life, Rejuvenate, Freedom Plus and Cypress, for great results. It is nice to dilute and use for a full body massage. **Companion Oils**: When the heart is stressed use Rose, Grateful, Guardian, Utopia, Calming, Confidence, Love, or Peacemaker.

CITRUS PLUS:
Contains – Orange, Lemon, Grapefruit, Mandarin, Bergamot, Tangerine, Lime (Distilled), & Vanilla.
This combination is invigorating and was formulated to assist the feeling of well-being. It is beneficial for digestive problems, cleans the lymphatic system, is a liver tonic, improves circulation, fights infectious diseases, and assists nervousness, anxiety and depression. It refreshes a tired mind, awakens creativity, gives confidence, inspires harmony, and promotes self-awareness. Citrus Plus balances emotions either relaxing or stimulating as needed, inspiring harmony, awakening creativity, and restoring joy.

It is beneficial used for water retention, breaking down cellulite fat pockets, inflammation, digestion, viral infections, reduces fevers, flu, strengthens the liver, and assists muscle tone and intestinal spasms. It assists circulation in the extremities, supports the lymphatic and nervous systems, stimulates the brain, and helps concentration. It brings back childlike energy, calms anger, frustration, reduces stress, depression, resentment, relieves anxiety, is

uplifting and stabilizes a person in a shaky emotional state assisting in reopening the heart to heal.

The Citrus Plus offers all-natural, cleansing abilities with potent compounds. It is great for being used as a house-hold cleanser and disinfectant that can be diluted with water. It is an ideal disinfectant that is safe for both the family and pets, has a sweet fresh citrus aroma that is elevating, uplifting, and soothing. This fragrance is enjoyed by children and makes a wonderful disinfectant when diffused because of its ability to kill airborne pathogens, boosts, and strengthen the immune system.

Traditional Application: apply on the ears, heart, and wrists. Wear as a perfume or use in a massage or relaxing bath. **Companion Oils:** Serenity, Love, Grateful, and Joyful. **Caution**: Citrus oils are phototoxic and can be irritating to the skin.

CONFIDENCE:
Contains - Rosewood, Spruce, Frankincense and Blue Tansy
It assists in overcoming fear and opposition so we can stand tall during adversity. It builds self-esteem, gives the confidence and courage to speak your truth, brings a feeling of calmness, peace, and relaxation. It has been found to be beneficial in assisting the alignment of the physical structure of the body, repairing injuries of the spine, and is sometimes called "the chiropractor in the bottle". Use Confidence to bring electrical energies, within the body, back into harmony. It is grounding, improves balance, coordination, relieves stress, and nervousness.

Traditional Application: on the wrists, massaged along the spine, and the throat from neck to thymus. When you feel brain tired, balance the brain by rubbing a drop of Confidence on the temples. To assist in keeping you balanced and aligned, rub a few drops on the bottom of your feet each morning. **Companion Oil:** To get the best use of all your oil, first use Confidence on the bottom of the feet to balance. All oils work well with Confidence.

CREAMSICLE:
Contains – Orange and Vanilla
It makes a wonderful nerve sedative, balances the emotions of anger, frustration, calms, awakens creativity, eases tension, it brings warm feelings of joy, and gratitude. It is a favorite for children.
Traditional Application: apply on wrists, ears, back of neck, on legs, and diffuse. **Companion Oils:** Citrus Plus, Peaceful Moments, Love, Forgiveness, Grateful, Magnify, and Peacemaker.

DNA REPAIR:
Contains – Ylang Ylang Extra, Cedarwood, Frankincense, Rose, Elemi, Cinnamon, Cypress, Sandalwood, Helichrysum italicum, Myrtle, Hyssop, Myrrh, and Peppermint
These oils were specifically selected for the three main classes of compounds that occur naturally in the plants and have the intelligence and capability to benefit our bodies. It clears the receptor sites of the cells allowing the cells to communicate, improve body functions, and elevate one's mood. It has the ability to erase or reprogram miswritten codes in the DNA. This makes DNA Repair very effective in releasing stuck or deep, hidden negative emotions, and in purging confused thoughts of anger or despair. It is neuro-balancing, uniting the head and heart allowing us to release past hurts, creating a sense of well-being, and love. It leads to greater spiritual insight, generosity, and eases fears.

DNA Repair instills peace, assists in adding balance, and control to our lives. It motivates us to move forward, assists with transitions or changing course in life, eases the feelings of loss, heals emotions, creates a feeling of security, and is grounding. It is uplifting, assists with personal growth, encourages compassion, and enhances the subconscious. It is beneficial for fatigue, infection, inflammation, digestive disorders, bronchitis, soothing to the nerves, a heart tonic, and supports all systems of the body.

Traditional Application: apply seven drops on the bottom of the feet to assist when emotionally stuck. Apply on the ears, forehead, wrists, temples, back of the neck, in a massage, as a perfume, or after-shave. **Companion Oils:** Angel Assist, Guardian, Uplifting, Confidence, and Peacemaker.

DREAMTIME:
Contains - Sandalwood, Patchouli, Ginger Root, Jasmine, and Petitgrain
It assists in the processing of emotional pain and ancestral ties during sleep through our dreams by opening the mind and enhancing the dream-state. It protects from negative influences that try to steal our vision and goals. Dreamtime assists in locking our goals and dreams into the mind so we dream with intent. It is soothing and relaxing.

Traditional Application: rub across the forehead, eyebrows, behind the ears, on the temples, and throat energy center at the base of neck. Put under your nose or on your pillow for dream awareness. It is used for mediation and sweat lodges. For a soothing bath add eight drops to your bath water. It is nice to diffuse during sleep or meditation.
Companion Oils: Magnify, Passion for Life, Angel Assist, Meditation, Uplifting, Harmony, and In The Moment. **Comments:** If bad dreams come, keep using the oil for something in your subconscious needs to process. See the dreams you want in your life, bring them from your mind to your heart, and commit to make them come true.

ENVISION:
Contains - Orange, Rose Geranium, Sage, and Spruce
It balances the emotions, assists in overcoming acute fear, emotional crises, depression, extreme moodiness, abuse, and hurt. It is consoling, eases anxiety and tension, brings joy to the heart, renews faith in the future, and maintains the emotional fortitude to achieve one's dreams. It inspires the imagination and assists in the awareness of all that is going on around us. Healing occurs in the presence of awareness. It keeps us focused which is necessary to release the hurt of the past so we are free to move on.

Traditional Application: apply around the ankles,

on the wrists, temples, across shoulders, in a full body massage, or add to bath water. Diffusing this oil may assist in reaching your dreams and goals. **Companion Oils:** Dreamtime, Love, Angel Assist, Grateful, Magnify, Prosperity, and Forgiveness.

EUPHORIA:
This unique blend is much like the seasons of the year. Each season contains their uniqueness yet adds variety and enjoyment to the year. This too, is the wonderment of Euphoria. From batch to batch it is never the same yet it will always be a wonderful surprise to experience.

EXODUS:
Contains – Frankincense, Cinnamon, Cassis, Hyssop, Myrrh, Galbanum, Spikenard, and Calamus
It assists circulation, strengthens the heart, endocrine, and nervous systems, and is an immune system builder. It promotes physical energy, is effective against colds, flu, fevers, asthma (clears the lungs), fungus, inflammation, parasites, viruses, infections, bacteria, tropical infections, and is a tonic for the digestive system. It is uplifting, calms restlessness, nervous fatigue, strengthens the mind, and supports the whole body.

Traditional Application: use the Vita Flex technique and apply to the back, along the spine, and on the bottoms of the feet. **Companion Oils:** Oregano, Peppermint, Ravintsara, Rejuvenation, Fortify, Spice Traders, and Freedom Plus.

FAITH:
Contains – Blue Tansy, Roman Chamomile, Ylang Ylang Extra, Lime, Mandarin, Lavender, and Rose.
Use when a little encouragement is needed to assist in dissolving emotional blocks that hinder personal growth. It gives the heart courage, helps ease anxiety, and diminishes depression. It stabilizes emotions, assisting in recovering from stress related conditions, promoting patience and peace, calms worries enabling one to have faith to move forward with life. It was created to inspire and spur ones

creativity bringing balance and harmony to the body. Good to use when making and setting new goals.

Because faith and fear cannot be present at the same time, when the body is calmed, out of stress or fear we can be open to make the changes needed. It is relaxing and soothing to the nervous system, and helps produce positive feelings of confidence. When applied to the throat area it may assist in expressing ones true feelings. It is stimulating and elevating to the mind creating a sense of well-being. When faith enters fear flees.

Traditional Application: across the forehead and temples, massage the ears, the back of the neck, over the heart, liver area, or on the wrists. **Companion Oils:** Confidence, Grateful, Love, Rose Blend, Angel Assist, and DNA Repair.

FIRST AID:
Contains – Cinnamon, Peppermint, Spearmint, Lime, Orange, and Lavender
This blend was formulated to assist circulation, strengthen the heart, the endocrine and nervous systems. It is beneficial against viruses, bacteria, parasites, inflammation, spasms, and fungus. It is an immune stimulant, antiseptic, and cools a fever or warms chills. It is beneficial for flu, coughs, cold, sore throat, congestion, headache, muscular aches and pains, stomach cramps, and intestinal spasms. First Aid is good for maintenance, relieving listlessness, depression, promotes physical energy, and refreshes a tired mind.

Traditional Application: beneficial when applied to the bottom of the feet and along the spine using the Vita Flex method. Massage into areas for sore muscles or stomach cramps. **Companion Oils:** Fortify, Birch, Ravintsara, Nerve Repair, Oregano, Thyme, Rejuvenate, Freedom Plus, Pine, and Pain EZ. **Caution:** It may be hot for sensitive skin.

FOCUS:
Contains - Rosemary, Peppermint, Holy Basil, Basil, and Cardamom

Focus provides an aroma that is clarifying and energizing, enhancing alertness, clear thought, dispelling confusion, awakens the brain, and sharpens the mental processes. It clears the head, improves concentration, memory, assists poor circulation, mental fatigue, strengthens the mind, and clears focus to handle the task at hand. Use for fainting, headaches, infections, stimulates for the nerves, and reduces stress.

Researchers found when peppermint oil was inhaled it increased the mental accuracy of the students being tested by 28%. Focus is good to use when studying and then smell it again while being tested on the material studied. It has been known to help with recall, may boost low energy, and keep someone from going into shock.

Traditional Application: across the forehead, the back of the neck, temples, and wrists. Put one drop in the palm of your hand, rub hands together, cup over your nose, and inhale deeply for a brain wake-up call. **Companion Oils:** Confidence, Brain Power, Passion for Life, Nerve Repair, and Magnify.

FORGIVENESS:
Contains - Spearmint, Myrtle, Ravintsara, Geranium, Hyssop, Rose Blend, Lavender, Clary Sage, Sage, Vetiver, and Lemon

It was formulated to assist in letting go of the negative past and increasing the desire to change. It brings an immediate emotional release of feelings of anger, fear, frustration, loss, despair, and feeling overwhelmed. It assists in bringing back love, peace, happiness, and a childlike innocence that opens one up to hope and beauty. It sooths lack of composure, is deeply relaxing, and strengthens the aura around the body. Use it when there is a conflict in thoughts and intellect. It helps deal with the energy that is blocking the changes you desire. As you find the block, release the energy behind the belief that created it, you are free to discover and create your own magnificence.

Forgiveness balances the central nervous system and decongests the liver. What you see, hear, feel, have, and are, depends on whether or not you have an attitude of forgiveness or non-forgiveness. Forgiveness removes blame. When you have an attitude of forgiveness, you see people as friends, and they see you as a friend. It is your choice.

Traditional Application: apply one drop on each ear and massage around the entire ear. Other areas to apply Forgiveness are over the navel, solar plexus, across the forehead, on the temples, over the liver, and on the bottom of the feet. **Companion Oils:** Break Thru, In The Moment, Love, Utopia, Guardian, DNA Repair, Balance, and Calming.

FORTIFY:
Contains - Frankincense, Juniper Berry, Nutmeg, Holy Basil, Ravintsara, Rosemary, Oregano, Ginger, Blue Tansy, Black Cumin, Clove Bud, and Hyssop

Fortify was formulated to build, strengthen, and protect the body. It is an incredible immune builder strengthening the body against inflammation, tumors, infections, viruses, bacteria, fungus, and parasites. It fights the spread of contagious disease, is beneficial for liver and kidney problems, skin disorders, detoxifying and cleansing the body, assists against infectious mononucleosis, sinusitis, and lymph congestion.

Fortify benefits the respiratory, digestive, nervous, and circulatory systems. It supports the adrenals, increases energy, and assists in expelling catarrh beneficial for spasms, fevers, viruses, strengthens the vital centers of the body, and rejuvenates the system quickly. It is useful in protecting the home environment from disease, revives exhausted emotions, clears mental confusion and fatigue, improves memory, inspires the desire to achieve, and eases depression, anxiety, and stress.

Traditional Application: apply three drops on the thymus in a clockwise motion for 30 seconds and then stimulate the thymus by tapping. Apply to the jugular veins on each side of the neck. Massage along the spine using the Vita Flex technique. Putting a few drops on each foot in the morning may provide protection from chemicals in the environment. Use under the arms to assist in strengthening the immune system especially for young children. **Companion Oils:** Oregano, Thyme, Clove, Cinnamon Blend, Spice Traders, Exodus, Rejuvenate, and Freedom Plus.

FREEDOM:
Contains - Neem, Peppermint, Black Cumin, Helichrysum, and Black Pepper
In Africa the Neem tree has been known for centuries as "the tree that heals." It has its own distinct smell which may be offensive to some. For millions of people this tree has miraculous powers and they report having received help within minutes.

Freedom assists with colds, hepatitis, acne, allergies, hives, Bell's palsy, AIDS, bruises, cold sores, bee stings, diaper rash, dry skin, ear ache, fever, infections, inflammation, and indigestion. It assists with jock itch, psoriasis, scabies, lice, cuts, sprains, eczema, hypertension, chickenpox, hair loss, Candida, chronic fatigue, circulation, kidney problems, headaches, obesity, ulcers, hemorrhoids, heartburn, diabetes, dandruff, malaria, urinary tract infection, wrinkles, parasites, stress, and yeast infection. It is also known to keep fleas away.

Traditional Application: massage into sore muscles, joints, and other areas wherever needed. Neem has a smell you may need to get used to. Excellent used on the face at night time.
Companion Oils: Spice Traders, Exodus, Cinnamon, Ravintsara, Clove Bud, and Fortify.

FREEDOM PLUS:
Contains – Neem, Lemongrass, Peppermint, Black Cumin, Helichrysum, and Black Pepper
The lemongrass gives Freedom Plus a lemon smell that takes away the strong smell of the Neem. For millions of people the Neem Tree has brought miraculous healing powers and they report having received help within minutes. It contains the same oils as the Freedom except for the lemongrass which makes it excellent for regenerating connective tissue, and repairing ligaments.

To receive even greater benefits gently massage into arthritic areas, apply a hot wet compress over the area, then a plastic bag to keep things dry followed by a bath towel to keep the heat in. Leave on for 15 minutes while the Freedom Plus goes deeper into the area. Freedom Plus is beneficial for inflammation, indigestion, cold sores, bee stings, fevers, and infections. It has been known to keep fleas away.

Traditional Application: massage into sore muscles, joints, back, insect bites, and stings. It is always good to use a hot compress when applying to sore muscles. **Companion Oils:** Pain EZ, Relief, Sports Pro, and Soothing Relief. **Caution:** This oils may burn sensitive skin areas such as the face or a baby's bottom.

GENTLE HEALER:
Contain - Rosemary, Tea Tree, Clove Buds and Helichrysum italicum
It was primarily formulated to assist with building and regenerating connective tissue from damage or injury. It assists with cuts, bruises, skin rashes, scrapes, and insect bites. It is a general tonic, beneficial for spasms viruses, bacteria, infections (especially useful against staph and strap), fungus, inflammation, parasites, and is a wonderful pain reliever.

It is beneficial for the respiratory, endocrine, and immune systems. Gentle Healer assists poor circulation, stimulates liver cell function, mental fatigue, and is an energy stimulant, controls mood swings, clears negative thoughts and memories. It is uplifting, arouses ambition and drive, inspires the desire to achieve, strengthens will power, and gives a sense of healing, protection, and courage. It has been used to assist animals with deep flesh wounds.

Traditional Application: apply topically to injured area. For earaches put a drop on a cotton ball and place in the ear. **Companion Oils:** Freedom Plus, Tea Tree, Peppermint, Rejuvenate, Spice Traders, and Fortify.

GROUNDING:
Contains - Vetiver, Frankincense, Lavender and Cedarwood

In research tests it was establish that the oils in this blend were definitely beneficial for those with ADD and ADHD. The Vetiver was the most effective showing it helped 100% of the test cases. Since all the oils noted some benefit when used singularly we have noted the benefits were enhanced when they were blended, it's the synergistic effect. It balances and regulates the Central Nervous System, assists in clearing the lymph system, is deeply relaxing, calming and healing for emotional wounds. It fortifies the mind, clears mental cobwebs, increases oxygen, and stimulates the cells' restorative power. It has been known to assist in calming angry situations.

Traditional Application: Effective massaged around the toes both top and bottom, on the brain stem, temples, and across the forehead. Apply several times during the day and put a few drops on the pillow at night. Put a few drops on a tissue and have it close where you can smell it when you start to feel out of control. **Companion Oils:** Basil, Peppermint, Rosemary, Spruce, Helichrysum italicum, Vetiver, and Focus.

GRATEFUL:
Contains – Ylang Ylang Extra, Roman Chamomile, and Rose

This is a wonderful blend to assist in focusing with gratitude on the blessings we have received. It will help move through the negative experiences faster by looking for the good things we have learned from the experience. It eases anxiety, dispels anger, gives patience, calms the mind, assists in balancing the equilibrium and heart functions, helps release past hurts, and brings a feeling of love.

When we are able to see past the negative and appreciate more fully the opportunities we have been given we move to a higher level of love and understanding in our life. Our experiences assist us in taking a closer look at our emotions, to re-evaluate what is going on in our life and make

needed changes. Grateful assists in overcoming emotional coldness, relationships, brings balance, and harmony to the body. The two things you can do in this life that will bring more joy to you is to forgive and be grateful.

Traditional Application: on the ears, forehead, temples, wrists, heart, and liver. **Companion Oils:** Love, Balance, Magnify, Peacemaker, Overcome, Uplifting, Hope, Present Moments, Faith, and Passion for Life.

GUARDIAN:
Contains – Spruce, Rosewood, Geranium, Hyssop, Angelica Root, Ylang Ylang Extra, Bergamot, Sandalwood, Myrrh, Rose Otto, Melissa and White Lotus absolute

Guardian was formulated to create a feeling of being in a special place with protection around you. It wards off the bombardment of negative energy, increases the aura around the body bringing balance, and harmony. It promotes gentleness, peace, is very soothing to the nerves relieving nervous tension, and stress. It reopens the heart center for loving feelings, awakens awareness, motivates you to move forward in life feeling safe, loved, and protected.

Traditional Application: across the shoulders, temples, forehead, ears, wrists, and solar plexus. **Companion Oils:** Balance, Love, Magnify, Faith, Mountain Retreat, Grateful, Uplifting, Peaceful Moments, Confidence, and Passion for Life.

HAIR SUPPORT:
Contains – Rosemary, Ravintsara, Ylang Ylang Extra, Cedarwood, Holy Basil, and Sage

It was formulated to strengthen and support healthy hair growth. It is beneficial against hair loss, dandruff, and improves circulation to the scalp when massaged into the hair. Hair Support is excellent for skin infections, promotes new cell growth, and is calming and soothing to the nervous system. It assists in giving the mind strength and clarity, is a general stimulant, beneficial as a restorative and strengthens the immune system. Dilute if necessary.

Traditional Application: at night massage a small amount into the scalp and leave on all night. After massaging the scalp apply a hot towel treatment to help push the oils into the skin. **Companion Oils:** Baldness may be due to fear, tension, and not trusting the process of life. Use oils such as Confidence, Serenity, Peacemaker, Calming, or Frankincense to calm and then affirmations at least ten times when you first wake up and before sleep. Good affirmations to use would be – "I am safe. I love and approve of myself. I trust life."

HOPE:
Contains – Lemongrass, Myrrh, Spruce, Juniper Berry, Ylang Ylang Extra, Orange, Lemon, Roman Chamomile, Petitgrain, and Melissa
It assists in bringing us out of denial, removes resistance, allows us to believe in ourselves and encourages us to do our best at all times. It awakens within us our ability to make transitions in our life to move on to achieve greater things. It assists in supporting the body mentally to give us hope and the assurance we have the ability to achieve. This formula reconnects us with a feeling of strength and grounding, removes blocks, and instills a positive outlook. Hope assists in bringing to reality what we desire. It has been known to relieve feelings of being down and discouraged bringing hope when feeling lost or abandoned.

Traditional Application: apply on ears, over the heart, temples, back of the neck, on wrists and solar plexus. For suicidal thoughts, apply to ears, over heart, and wrists. **Companion Oils:** Forgiveness, Love, Angel Assist, Grateful, Balance, DNA Repair, Guardian, Faith, and Peacemaker.

HORMONE BALANCE:
Contains - Vetiver, Clary Sage, Sandalwood, Bergamot, Petitgrain, Cinnamon Bark, Neroli, Lemon, and Orange
It assists in overcoming depression, anxiety, and is grounding in order to help us deal logically and peacefully with reality. When used in times of personal challenges it exerts a balancing influence. It is deeply relaxing, very calming, supporting in

cases of low self-confidence, and fear. It opens the heart center for healing emotional wounds, loving feelings, and gratitude. It brings joy, harmony and removes negative programming from the cells of the body to help us focus in the moment releasing resentment, touchiness, and grudges. It may assist in balancing hormones, alleviating pre-menstrual and menstrual cramps, discomfort, and other associated problems.

Traditional Application: massage across lower back, lower abdomen, and apply a hot compress. Apply around the ankles, on the ears, and under the nose for emotional support. **Companion Oils:** Geranium, DNA Repair, Peacemaker, Citrus Plus, Peaceful Moments, Balance, Calming, Uplifting, and Grateful.

IN THE MOMENT:
Contains – Vanilla Bourbon, Jasmine absolute, Neroli, Rose Otto, Mandarin, Bergamot, Lemon, Cedarwood, and Sandalwood
It assists in healing the body by removing the negative programming from the cells and bringing the mind, body, and spirit into balance. It assists to focus in the present moment. Yesterday is gone, tomorrow is unknown, and all you have is the present moment.

When you allow the body to release the past that is no longer serving you in a positive and progressive way you can heal. Only when you are consciously living in the moment can you release the negative past. It assists in calming anger, dissolving emotional blocks, stress, anxiety, depression, and nervous tension by creating a sense of well-being, self-confidence, and joy. It contains essential oils that are excellent for all skin conditions.

Traditional Application: it makes a beautiful perfume. Rub over the heart, on the ears, neck, thymus, and temples. Massage a few drops across the forehead, on the wrists or dilute and use in a full body massage. Add eight to ten drops to your bath water for a relaxing bath. Very beneficial to use on the ears and under the nose to bring yourself into the moment so you can deal with emotions from the past. When you look at the past emotion see the good you have learned from them and express gratitude for the experience. **Companion Oils:** Grateful, Confidence, Break Thru, Angel Assist, Balance, Faith, Calming, and Peacemaker.

JASMINE BLEND:
Contains – Jasmine and FCO
This is an affordable way to experience Jasmine. It is beneficial for stress, apathy, anxiety, nervous exhaustion, depression, indifference, listlessness, energy, confidence and all skin care. It assists with hoarseness, laryngitis, lethargy (abnormal drowsiness), menstrual problems, impotence, frigidity and uterine disorders. Jasmine may ease labor pains and encourage contractions, assists the speed of the expulsion of the afterbirth and overall recovery from giving birth, relieves postnatal depression, assists in stimulating milk production, and tones the uterus.

Jasmine Blend strengthens the male reproductive system, relieves discomfort of an enlarged prostate gland, and is beneficial for inflammation. It spurs creativity, inspires artistic expression, awakens intuition, awakens an appreciation of beauty in the world, and dissolves emotional blocks that hinder personal growth.

Traditional Application: apply across the forehead, in a massage, bath, and on the ears. **Caution:** can stimulate menstruation. It should be avoided during pregnancy until childbirth is imminent. **Companion Oils:** Passion for Life, Uplifting, Balance, Magnify, Grateful, and Guardian.

JOYFUL:
Contains - Orange, Spruce, Frankincense, Myrrh, Pine, Peppermint, Fir, and Cinnamon Bark
It was created to enhance the feelings and memories of the Holiday Season, and brings the desire to recapture the joyful moments. It balances the emotions, relaxing or stimulating as needed, awakening creativity, inspiring harmony, and promoting self-awareness. It is grounding, calming,

uplifting, assists to motivate you to move forward, and to eliminate blocked personal growth. Joyful improves concentration, energizes, and relieves mental fatigue. This blend protects against airborne viruses, and bacteria when diffused it is a pleasant air purifier and fragrance for the home.

Traditional Application: wear as perfume, cologne, on the wrists, and feet. Put on pine cones, cedar chips, and logs to burn in the fireplace. It is excellent to use in potpourri all year round. Add 30 drops to eight ounces of plain bath gel to protect the skin from viruses and bacteria. **Companion Oils:** Confidence, Balance, Angel Assist, Citrus Plus, Peacemaker, Mountain Retreat, Uplifting and Grateful.

LOVE:
Contains - Lemon, Orange, Rose Geranium, Bergamot, Mandarin, Ylang Ylang Extra, and Rose
Love was formulated to bring joy into our lives. When inhaled it brings back memories of being loved, being held, sharing loving times, and feelings. It will assist in opening our lives where perhaps we have shut down to love, to receiving love, or to self-love. When there is grief the adenoids and the adrenals shut down Love may assist in opening these glands. It assists in overcoming grief, forgiving others, and letting go of negative experiences. What may have seemed like obstacles are no longer viewed as obstacles but opportunities to learn and grow from.

Traditional Application: rub over the heart, ears, on the back of the neck, thymus, temples, across the forehead, and on the wrists. It is nice to use as a perfume or after-shave. Add to bath water or use as a compress. Wonderful diluted in carrier oil for a full body massage. It creates a frequency of love, the true source of all healing. **Companion Oils:** Angel Assist, DNA Repair, Uplifting, Grateful, Guardian, Balance, Peacemaker, Faith, and Mountain Retreat. **Caution:** It contains photosensitive oils so keep the applied area away from direct sunlight.

MAGNIFY:
Contains - Black Pepper, Bergamot, Holy Basil, Lemon, Orange, Lavender, Rose Otto, Roman Chamomile, Frankincense, German Chamomile, and Ylang Ylang Extra

It assists in being single minded with our heart feeling the same as our mind is thinking. This way we can rise above negative emotions and magnify our life's purpose. It builds self-esteem and a stronger desire for reaching goals. It may be beneficial to diffuse while goal setting. It assists in maintaining focus and creates a space for prayer and meditation. It helps overcome self-defeating behaviors such as procrastination, self-pity, feelings of abandonment, rejection, and betrayal.

Traditional Application: apply to the wrists, temples, across the forehead, on the crown of the head, across the shoulders, and neck. It is nice to use for an uplifting massage, diffused, or worn as a perfume. **Companion Oils:** Angel Assist, Faith, Calming, Love, Peaceful Moments, Grateful, Balance, and Passion for Life.

MEDITATION:
Contains – Orange, Spruce, Frankincense, Spikenard, Pine, Myrrh, Peppermint, Fir, and Cinnamon Bark

The oils in this blend are recognized for inspiring harmony, increasing spiritual and psychic awareness, strengthening beliefs, enhancing visualization, awakening creativity, and will assists in eliminating block personal growth. It slows breathing, acts as a sedative yet elevating to the mind, and provides support and balance to the heart, endocrine, and nervous systems.

Meditation assists in releasing stuck emotions, healing emotional wounds, dispelling pride, and bringing feelings of gratitude, generosity, and a deep inner peace. It is mentally grounding, calms anxiety, indecision, assists in overcoming fear of the future, and motivates one to move forward. It is calming and relaxing assisting one to reach a state of meditation.

Traditional Application: apply across the back of the neck, forehead, temples, and breathe deeply.
Companion Oils: Rose, In The Moment, Faith, Peaceful Moments, and Dreamtime. **Caution:** this oil **should not be used** when you are driving.

MELISSA BLEND:
Contains – Melissa and FCO

It is very soothing, relieves tension, and is, with Rose and Neroli, one of the major oils of the heart energy center. It is beneficial for depression, spasms and powerful for viruses. It is beneficial for the nerves, as an insect repellant, tonic for sore muscles and fatigue. Melissa calms circulation, strengthens and slows the heart, lowers blood pressure, and eases palpitations due to unusual stimulation, fear, or excitement.

It is beneficial for cold sores, herpes, fungal infections, asthma, insomnia, migraines, nervousness, neurasthenia, anxiety, wounds (stops blood flow), colds (with headache), chronic coughs, rapid breathing, shingles, emotional shock, and grief. Melissa assists in dealing with past issues, dispels fear, grief, and anger. It is uplifting bringing acceptance and understanding.

Traditional Application: apply on the wrists, forehead and on the feet. It is beneficial if added to salad dressing or a drop under the tongue.
Companion Oils: Exodus, Rejuvenate, Freedom Plus, Confidence, and Fortify.

MIGRAINE RELIEF:
Contains – Basil, Marjoram, Lavender, Peppermint, Helichrysum gymnocephalium, Roman Chamomile, and Helichrysum italicum

It is a blend of oils that synergistically provide you with nearly miraculous relief from inflammation and associated pain. It is calming as it eases nervous tension, stress, and poor circulation. Migraine Relief is uplifting, stimulates the regeneration of new cells, and eases anxiety, worries, and fear.

It assists with headaches, migraines, balances extremes in emotions, and provides comfort during times of grief. It is beneficial for lowering blood pressure, relaxes the mind, and assists with muscular aches, pain, and stiffness. Migraine Relief assists with spasms, fatigue, infections, sprains, fluid retention, cramps, depression, and is a sedative.

Traditional Application: apply a few drops topically to the back of the neck, across the forehead, and on the temples. **Companion Oils:** Nerve Repair, True Blue, Lavender, Clove Buds, Birch, Sports Pro, Soothing Relief, Freedom Plus, and Relief.

MOUNTAIN RETREAT:
Contains - Spruce, Fir, Pine, Cedarwood, Ylang Ylang Extra, and Frankincense
It is grounding, stimulating, elevating, and opening to bring about a balance of emotions. Mountain Retreat is calming, relaxing, and soothing to the nerves. It dispels anger, frustration, poor self-esteem, anxiety, and depression. It stimulates circulation, clears mental cobwebs, balances the equilibrium, heart functions, and enhances relationships. It is known to increase spirituality and self-control giving a feeling of "I can do it." It assists us in feeling safe to set goals, to dream, and gives us strength and courage to manifest them in our lives. The conifer oils were traditionally used by the North American Indians to symbolically represent a protective umbrella for the earth bringing energy in from the universe.

Traditional Application: apply to the solar plexus, brain stem, crown of the head, back of the neck, across the shoulders, behind and on the ears, thymus, and wrists. Diffuse or wear as a perfume. **Companion Oils:** Confidence, Peacemaker, Faith, Prosperity, Serenity, DNA Repair, and Balance.

NEROLI BLEND:
Contains – Neroli and FCO
This is an affordable way to experience the many benefits of Neroli. The Egyptian people used Neroli for healing the mind, body, and spirit. It seems to bring everything into focus at the moment. It is beneficial for scars, stretch marks, thread veins, mature and sensitive skin, and tones the complexion. It is beneficial for poor circulation, wrinkles, palpitations, diarrhea (chronic), colic, flatulence, spasm, nervous dyspepsia, anxiety, depression, nervous tension, shock, stress related conditions, and emotional problems.

Traditional Application: after washing the face and neck, apply a few drops night and morning. Wonderful used as a perfume, in a massage, on the forehead, ears, or in a bath. One drop under the tongue assists with depression and anxiety. **Companion Oils:** Balance, Grateful, Utopia, Love, Hormone Balance, Forgiveness, and Guardian.

NERVE REPAIR:
Contains – Basil, Helichrysum italicum, Peppermint, and Marjoram
These oils assist in repairing damaged nerves, stimulates circulation, eases inflammation swelling, and cramps. It works on the parasympathetic nerves, is a great pain reliever, infection fighter, and helps in healing and repairing connective tissue that has been damaged. It is restorative, a stimulant for nerves, and assists in the regenerates of new cells. It is beneficial for nervous tension, stress, and very soothing to the nerves by just breathing it in.

Traditional Application: massage into the area where the nerves have been damaged, apply a cold compress, and relax for at least 15 minutes. For an earache apply a couple of drops to cotton and place in the ear. Massage on the shoulders, neck, and across the forehead for nervous stress and tension. For a fever add a few drops of carrier oil, massage the head, and back. **Companion Oils:** Basil, Spruce, True Blue, Relief, Freedom Plus, Fortify, and Confidence.

OVERCOME:
Contains - Rosewood, Grapefruit, Holy Basil, Frankincense, Bay Leaf, Indian Peppermint, Galbanum, Jasmine, Rose Otto, Hyssop, Roman Chamomile, and Pink Lotus absolute
It was formulated to create a feeling of humility and the ability to overcome the fear that sometimes stops us from being the best we can. It assists us from

drowning in negativity, is strengthening, stabilizing, and uplifting. It creates a sense of well-being in the whole body. It promotes alertness, clarity, and is elevating to the mind.

Overcome is balancing to the emotions, relaxing emotional links to the past, and healing emotional wounds. It assists in eliminating blocked personal growth such as dispelling anger, pride, and feelings of inferiority. It releases anxiety, stress, depression, is calming, and relaxing to the nerves. It promotes peace, confidence, spurs creativity, and helps a person express their true feelings. It helps find the special place where our own healing may begin.

Traditional Application: rub over the heart, neck, temples, across the forehead, over the solar plexus, for a massage, or diffused. **Companion Oils:** Love, Balance, Confidence, Break Thru, Forgiveness, Grateful, Faith, DNA Repair, and Guardian.

PAIN EZ:
Contains – Lemongrass, Birch and Peppermint
Pain EZ was formulated to assist in reducing pain and stimulating quicker healing. It is excellent when used for inflammation, repairing ligaments, headaches, and circulation. Beneficial for arthritis, sprains, bruises, pulled muscles, and other unbroken skin injuries with pain.

Traditional Application: massage into the areas where there is soreness and pain. Apply a hot wet compress to the area, cover with a plastic bag and then a towel in order to keep the heat in. Keep covered for about 15 minutes. **Companion Oils:** Basil, Helichrysum, Spruce, Relief, Freedom Plus, True Blue, Soothing Relief, and Sports Pro.

PASSION FOR LIFE:
Contains - Tangerine, Bergamot, Jasmine grandiflorum absolute, Rose Geranium, Citronella, Helichrysum italicum, Vetiver, Frankincense, and Holy Basil
It was formulated to eliminate blocked personal growth, dissolve emotional blocks, and activate the right brain arousing appreciation for beauty, spurring creativity, awakening intuition, and enhancing the subconscious. It is used for relieving emotional grief, stress, and letting go of the negative past. It brings about a sense of peace, restores joy, loving feelings, and overcomes acute fear. Passion is a fire within. It is the heartfelt energy that flows through us, not from us. It fills our heart when we allow it to and it inspires others when we share it. It is like sunlight flowing through a doorway that we have just opened. Our passion was always there, it just needed to be accepted and embraced.

Passion for Life reminds us that we are meant to be purposeful, positive, and passionate. We feel this when we listen to and accept our calling in life. We feel it as inspiration when we open the door of resistance and let it in. It awakens in us an optimistic attitude. It is extremely uplifting, refreshing, and arousing. Remember a lack of passion is at the foundation of hopelessness and failure. This may be a beneficial essential oil to assist you through these times in awakening your passion for life.

Traditional Application: it may be used for massage, perfume, behind the ears, on the wrists, apply under the nose, across the shoulders, and across the forehead. It contains some beneficial oils for skin problems. It is wonderful to diffuse. **Companion Oils:** Love, Confidence, Overcome, Magnify, Brain Power, In the Moment, and Faith.

PEACEFUL MOMENTS:
Contains – Frankincense (India), Lime (distilled), Orange, Balsam of Peru, Sandalwood, Patchouli, Blue Tansy, White Grapefruit, and Ylang Ylang Extra
This was formulates to assist us in being at peace with what is going on around us. It dispels anger, eases anxiety, frustration, and nervous tension, assists in healing emotional wounds, stress, depression, fear, grief, and obsessions. It is beneficial for poor circulation, digestion, fevers, inflammation, muscle tone, water retention, bacteria, parasites, fungus, viruses, infections, and assists with wound healing, is tissue regenerative, a liver

tonic, and stimulates the lymphatic system. It is grounding, strengthens and integrates energy to all areas of the body, calms worries, uplifting relaxing, very soothing, brings love, inspires harmony, improves self-esteem, gives patience, and peace.

Traditional Application: apply on ears, over the heart, temples, back of the neck, on wrists, and solar plexus. For suicidal thoughts, apply to the rim of the ears, on the face next to the ear flap, over the heart, and wrists. **Companion Oils:** Rose, Faith, Grateful, Love, Guardian, Peacemaker, and Angel Assist.

PEACEMAKER:
Contains – Litsea Cubeba, Lime, Mandarin, Pink Grapefruit, Tangerine, Sandalwood, and Ylang Ylang Extra
This particular blend is cheering, uplifting, stimulating, and balancing. Peacemaker is beneficial in bringing back child-like energy, and signifies the inner child. It gives confidence, carries oxygen to the brain, helps remove negative programming from the cells, and calms the nerves. It assists in balancing the equilibrium and heart functions, supports all the systems of the body, acts as a general tonic assisting with inflammation, and infections. It is beneficial for meditation, relieving resentment, depression, dispelling anger, anxiety, fear, stress, guilt, and relieving grief. It is refreshing, enhances relationships, and brings peace.

Traditional Application: on the ears, forehead, wrists, and temples, back of the neck, in a massage, as a perfume or after-shave. Enjoy experimenting with all the different ways to use Peacemaker such as in your bath water or diffusing. **Companion Oils:** Angel Assist, Love, Peaceful Moments, Guardian, Balance, Faith, Utopia, Confidence, Calming, Citrus Plus, Uplifting, and Lavender.
Scripture: "Blessed are the peacemakers."

PROSPERITY:
Contains - Orange, Spruce, Patchouli, Clove, Frankincense, Myrrh, Cinnamon Bark, Lemon, and Cypress
It was formulated to enhance magnetic energy and evoke the law of attraction through the magnetic field around us. By keeping our thoughts on what we do want, we create an electrical stimulation, and put out a frequency charge of abundance. It seems to attract prosperity in any area you focus your attention. Be careful what you think about because that is what you will attract an abundance of.

This particular formula contains very powerful oils that support the body against virus, bacteria, fungus, parasites, inflammation, and infections. It is elevating and opening bringing balance to the emotions. Prosperity supports the glandular, immune, respiratory, and nervous systems. It assists in recovery from stress-related conditions, sharpens the intellect, awakens awareness, improves concentration, promotes physical energy, strengthens, and assists in eliminating blocked growth, brings joy and gratitude into our life.

Traditional Application: since some of the oils in this blend are hot you may want to dilute before wearing on your wrists and feet. Put it on your checkbook and in your purse. To create more business, add a 15 ml. bottle to five gallons of paint, stir, and paint your workspace. When diffused it creates harmonic energy and opens the way for prosperity.

It's been helpful to use before going shopping for a specific item because it seems that item is always on sale. One lady told me that by diffusing Prosperity in her gift shop she was able to bring in more business. In Africa, I put six drops in a ¼ oz bottle of olive oil for a homeless man. He told me he always had enough to eat when he used the oil. I left him my whole bottle when I came home.
Companion Oils: Focus, Guardian, Grateful, Love, In The Moment, Balance, Magnify, and Mountain Retreat may be used first to help release the emotions that are stopping you from receiving abundance.
Scripture: "As a man thinketh in his heart, so is he." We are creating the kind of abundance we expect in all areas by our thoughts, actions, and words.

PURIFY:
Contains - Lemongrass, Rosemary, Tea Tree, Lavender, Myrtle, and Citronella
Purify was formulated especially for diffusing to kill airborne anaerobic bacteria, viruses, mold, fungus, neutralizes mildew, cigarette smoke, eliminate other noxious odors, and their problems. The aroma is very cleansing, beneficial in neutralizing poison from insect bites, spiders, bees, hornets, and wasps. It repels bugs, mice, assists in treating wounds and cuts, nervous exhaustion, respiratory conditions, poor circulation, assists the skin to heal, and regenerates connective tissue.

Traditional Application: apply to infected areas of the body. Diffuse when illness is in the home. Cycle the diffuser one hour on and two hours off. Diffuse in the office, barn, and garbage areas to stop the spread of infections and disease. Put 15 drops of Purify in a four-ounce spray bottle with water, shake, and spray around a hotel room - especially the mattress. To remove cigarette smoke from clothing, hang them in the bathroom and spray. Let the clothes hang overnight. When diffused in a freshly painted room, it has been known to eliminate paint fumes. **Companion Oils:** Lavender, Citronella, Peppermint, Rosemary, Tea Tree, Fortify, and Spice Traders.

REGENERATE:
Contains – Helichrysum italicum and Florah
The oil of Florah has traditionally been used for wounds, scars, and skin regeneration. The Helichrysum is extremely beneficial for any nerve problems, is an excellent pain reliever, and its properties for reducing inflammation exceed those of any other oil. It is beneficial for bruises, acne, eczema, sunburns, scaring, stimulates the regeneration of new cells, broken veins, stretch marks, and spots. It has virtually unlimited value in treating dermatitis and other skin disorders.

Traditional Application: apply topically to the affected areas. **Companion Oils:** Skin Care, Elemi, Myrrh, Frankincense, Rose, Geranium, Baby Soft, and Rejuvenate.

REJUVENATE:
Contains: Organic Lemon, Organic Orange, Organic Anise Seed, Organic Black Cumin, Peppermint, White Cedar, Clove Buds, Ginger Root, Ravintsara, Lemongrass, Spearmint, Organic Eucalyptus radiata, Cinnamon Bark, Lavender, Sandalwood, Organic Helichrysum italicum, and Frankincense
It is a general, all around maintenance oil, a powerful purifier, has a positive effect on all the systems of the body, and supports physical energy. It has been found to be effective against bacteria, viruses, parasites, inflammation, fungus, antiseptic, tumors, catarrh, and depression.

Rejuvenate is stimulating, strengthening, detoxifies the liver and kidneys, cleanses the blood, and stimulates red and white blood cell formation. It is very effective for nervous conditions, impaired digestion, water retention, pulmonary and lymphatic congestion, infections of any kind, poor circulation, allergies, skin disorders, and viruses.

It relieves mental fatigue, sharpens senses, and improves concentration and memory. It is beneficial for muscle cramps, aches, pains, spasms, swollen glands, strengthens the heart and assists in balancing the metabolism. It promotes health, assists in repairing damage done to the body through the use of nicotine and other addictive substances, and may curb the desire for them.

Traditional Application: on the back, in a full body massage using the Rejuvenation Technique and on the feet using the Vita Flex. I like to use ten to fifteen drops on my salad to add new zest to the dressing and assist my immune system. A drop under the tongue several times a day has been known to help those who want to stop smoking. One person reported using the Rejuvenate for a Brown Recluse spider bite with good results. **Companion Oils:** Support (for best results to stop smoking), Exodus, Spice Traders, Fortify, Freedom Plus, True Blue, Soothing Relief, Birch, Oregano, Cypress, Basil, and Frankincense.

RELIEF:
Contains – Helichrysum gymnocephalium, Birch, Clove Bud, Cypress, Peppermint, and Marjoram

It was formulated to assist in reducing pain and stimulating quick healing. It is beneficial for viruses, inflammation, bacteria, fungus, infections, spasms, and improves circulation. Relief has helped alleviate sciatica symptoms, relieve bone pain, assists muscle and joint discomfort. It is beneficial for sprains, bruises, fevers, respiratory problems, cramps, arthritis, sports injuries, stops bleeding, strengthens blood capillary walls, headaches, and rheumatism. It is a great pain reliever, assists in general healing, calms emotions, may provide comfort during times of grief, and stress related conditions.

Traditional Application: apply on location where there is discomfort or on the feet. **Companion Oils:** Cypress, Spruce, Basil, Birch, Wintergreen, Pine, Palmarosa, Freedom Plus, Sports Pro, True Blue, Soothing Relief, and Nerve Repair. **Caution:** Relief may sting when applied to an open wound.

RENEW:
Contains – Foraha, Rosemary, and Helichrysum italicum

It stimulates cell regeneration by increasing oxygen circulation to broken capillaries. Renew assists in repairing the damaged barrier function of the skin and helps in retaining moisture. When this barrier is left untreated, it causes dehydration and accelerated aging. It assists in improving the overall health of your skin and is especially beneficial for those living in a dry desert climate.

Traditional Application: wash face and apply to skin night and morning for best results.
Companion Oils: Geranium, Elemi, Skin Care, Frankincense, Roman Chamomile, and Spikenard.

RESP EZ:
Contains - Rosemary, Pine, and Lime

It assists with respiratory problems and goes along with the Breathe EZ. When an essential oil is used without seeing much of a benefit it is suggested you "try another oil." Resp EZ was added to our line because of the benefits noticed from this combination. It is a wonderful oil to use to stimulate circulation, fight colds, coughs, flu, sore throats, fevers, bronchitis, sinusitis, and strengthens the immune system. It has the ability to clear mucus quickly, is beneficial for nervous exhaustion, and assists stress related conditions.

Traditional Application: massage over the chest area, on the back (the lungs are actually closer to the back so remember this area), and apply a wet hot towel compress. Massage on the top and bottoms of the feet near the toe area. **Companion Oils:** Breathe EZ, Ravintsara, Rejuvenate, Exodus, Oregano (diluted), Fortify, and Hyssop.

ROSE BLEND:
Contains – Rose Otto and FCO

This is an affordable way to experience the wonderful benefits of Rose. It has an extraordinarily complex chemistry with over 300 known constituents. It enhances the frequency of every cell bringing balance and harmony to the body. Rose is said to be beneficial for depression, spasms, an antiseptic, bactericidal against strep, staph, E. coli, anthrax, diphtheria, diuretic, and hemostatic (anti-hemorrhagic). It is a nerve sedative, stomachic, and a tonic for the heart and liver.

Rose is known to be beneficial for hemorrhaging, infections, asthma, chronic bronchitis, tuberculosis, ulcers, sprains, assists conjunctivitis, herpes, skin disease, wrinkles, shingles, excellent for babies, radiation burns, thrush, eczema, gingivitis, wounds, broken capillaries, prevents scarring and revitalizes and rejuvenates dry, sensitive, or aging skin. Rose is stimulating and elevating to the mind, creates a sense of well-being, helps release past hurts, and brings a feeling of love.

Traditional Application: on the ears, forehead, temples, over the heart, or in a massage.
Companion Oils: Angel Assist, Love, Harmony, Peacemaker, Confidence, Grateful, and Faith.

SANDALWOODS:
Contains – Sandalwood from India, Indonesia, Australia, Africa, and the West Indies
It acts as a nerve sedative, urinary and pulmonary antiseptic, expectorant, stimulates the immune system, beneficial for spasms, fungus, infections, and depression. It assists and balances any skin type or condition (dry, aged, cracked, chapped, psoriasis, and eczema), wonderful for the scalp, increases water retention of collagen, increases circulation, and fat metabolism. Sandalwoods assist stress, insomnia, obsessions, fear, grief, feelings of isolation, aggression, and egocentric behavior. It assists in removing negative programming from the cells and is supportive in cases of low self-confidence.

Traditional Application: across the forehead, on the ears, back of the neck or in a massage.
Companion Oils: Neroli, Geranium, Skin Care, Breathe EZ, DNA Repair, Blossoms, Renew, and Circle of Life.

SERENITY:
Contains - Orange, Tangerine, Patchouli, Lime, Ylang Ylang Extra, Lavender, Blue Tansy, German Chamomile, and Citronella
Serenity promotes relaxation allowing us to relax so the blood can get up to the brain. It is grounding and integrates energy allowing us to visualize our goals and dreams more vividly and accurately. It assists in reducing depression, eases anxiety, stress, and tension. It brings joy to the heart, balances and stabilizes the emotions, gives patience, and calms worries. It is known to assist hyperactive children by creating serenity in their life. It has been found beneficial when used with children that have frequent nightmares. It may assist in curing the habit of smoking.

Traditional Application: on the wrists, ears, under the nose, back of the neck, add to bath water, and dilute with massage oil to rub on the back. For insomnia apply to navel, legs, and neck. Diffuse to assist in calming active or hard to manage children or adults. Diffusing has assisted people in coming

off drugs. It does miracles when traveling with small children; put 10 drops in a 2 oz spray bottle of water, shake, and spray anywhere you need to calm things down. **Companion Oils:** Lavender, Orange, Chamomile, Calming, Citrus Plus, Angel Assist, Love, Dreamtime, Creamsicle, Confidence, Uplifting, Peacemaker, and Grateful.

SKIN CARE:
Contains – Lavender, Frankincense, Carrot Seed, Neroli, Roman Chamomile, Rose Otto, in a base of Cucumber Seed
It was formulated to enhance the skin, benefits skin elasticity, and creates a youthful appearance. It assists in revitalizing, toning, rejuvenating dry, sensitive, or mature complexions. Beneficial when used for infections, inflammation, and circulation problems. It minimizes scarring, boosts immunity, increases cell growth assisting the skin to heal and rejuvenate. Skin Care is beneficial for skin ulcers, blemishes, scars, diaper rash, boils, dermatitis, eczema, ringworm, insect bites, psoriasis, wrinkles, thread veins, stretch marks, acne, sunburns, and bruises. It assists in bringing balance and harmony to the body, stabilizes the emotions and when applied over the throat, it may assist a person to express their true feelings. Rubbed into the belly regularly during pregnancy has been known to prevent stretch marks.

Traditional Application: apply to clean skin and gently massage upward. The emotion behind skin problems is fear, anxiety, or a feeling of being threatened. A good affirmation to use is "I lovingly protect myself with thoughts of joy and peace. The past is forgiven and forgotten. I am free in this moment. I feel safe to be me." Getting more omega-3 also benefits skin problems. **Companion Oils:** Confidence, Break Thru, Uplifting, Peacemaker, Balance, Peaceful Moments, and Renew.

SLIM & TRIM:
Contains - Pink Grapefruit, Lemon, Peppermint (India), Cinnamon Bark, Celery Seed, and Ginger.
It was formulated to assist in managing the appetite, stop cravings between meals, and impulsive eating.

Can you imagine looking at chocolate and not even feeling an urge to consume it simply because you don't feel the enticing? Food cravings can be both emotional and physical. When one is hungry we receive strong signals from the brain and various parts of the body letting us know we need nutrients. Generally with the urge we respond with eating and our body feels the rewards. Craving foods to satisfy an emotional can become a destructive habit.

It is important to make sure you are NOT eating foods that contain High Fructose Corn Syrup or MSG. They actually make your body have food cravings. They are now hidden in our processed foods under different names. It is best to eat less food and replace all manufactured and processed food with healthy all natural foods. Eating healthy foods in smaller amounts, using Slim & Trim and a regular exercise program will assist in getting to your ideal healthy weight.

A fit body offers a lifetime of vitality, energy, and helps to prevent degenerative diseases. It is done by eating less and having a regular work out. Slim & Trim is designed to help one manage appetite and food cravings between meals during the day. For best results add eight drops to a glass of water and drink between meals. You'll see even faster benefits if you take **Probiotics Plus** capsules along with your water.

The Slim & Trim also can lift moods and relax your stomach. It has a wonderful taste and gives a delicious flavor to water. It is great for supporting hydration with exercise. Another benefit of Slim & Trim is that it has zero calories, no artificial sweeteners, or colors.

It regulates body weight if used regularly, tones congested skin, assists eliminating water, stimulates circulation, dissolves accumulated uric acid in the joints, and decreases toxin built-up. It assists lymph drainage, cellulite, inflammation, liver congestion, digestive problems, tightens skin, and strengthens the glands. It assists with nervous disorders, stress, anxiety, infections, fatigue, cramps, and is stimulating but grounding.

Traditional Application: massage over the areas of cellulite concern and drink in water between meals. **Companion Oils:** Confidence, Pink Grapefruit, Citrus Plus, Envision, Faith, Forgiveness, In The Moment, and Love.

SOOTHING RELIEF:
Contains - Peppermint (India), Spruce, Wintergreen, Clove, Lemon, Vetiver, Helichrysum italicum, and Balsam Copaiba
Soothing Relief contains oils that synergistically produce greater benefits when combined. This formula offers soothing relief from pain, stress, fatigue, inflammation, regenerates new cell growth, increases oxygen, assists lymph drainage, repairs connective tissue, and stimulates liver cell function. Soothing Relief is beneficial for nerve problems, improves circulation, fights infection, assists digestion, has natural cortisone-like properties, restores depleted adrenal glands, and stimulates the thymus. It fights bacteria, infections, viruses, fungus, parasites, flu, muscle aches and pains, sprains, cramps, spasms, water retention, and reduces fevers. It is deeply relaxing, uplifting, and mentally grounding.

Traditional Application: apply on location where there is discomfort or on the feet. Beneficial used with a hot wet compress. **Companion Oils:** Basil, Birch, Helichrysum, True Blue, Relief, Sports Pro, Pain EZ, Freedom Plus, and Nerve Repair.

SPICE TRADERS:
Contains - Clove Bud, Cinnamon Bark, Lemon, Eucalyptus radiata, Thyme, Orange, Oregano, Nutmeg, Rosemary, Mandarin, and Ginger Root
It was formulated to strengthen the immune system and is powerful for all-around maintenance. It is beneficial against infections, viruses, bacteria, fungus, inflammation, parasites, spasms, and microbes. It is a general tonic and supports the nervous, respiratory, urinary, and circulatory systems. Spice Traders helps protect the body from the onset of malaria, flu, colds, and coughs. It assists in cooling a fever or warming chills, loosens and expels mucus, strengthens the digestive

functions, and aids the liver. It supports the adrenals, increases energy, and brings balance.

Spice Traders assists with dental infections, strep, gum disease, throat infections, teething, cold sores, canker sores, pneumonia, sinusitis, bronchitis, headaches, nervous fatigue, slivers, and splinters are pulled to surface. It is calming, promotes healing, and diffusing may inhibit the spread of infections. It contains oils considered anti-plague by the spice merchants living in England in the 16th century. They used various spices to protect themselves from the plague as they looted the bodies of the sick and dying.

Traditional Application: dilute one drop of Immune Strength with 5 to 15 drops of carrier oil. Massage the thymus, on the feet, and under the arms to strengthen the immune system. Apply diluted on the throat, around ears, stomach, and intestines. Diffuse periodically 30 minutes at a time when there is sickness in the home. **Companion Oils:** Fortify on the throat and Spice Traders on the feet and alternate the next day. Exodus, Cinnamon Blend, Clove Buds, Oregano, Thyme, Tea Tree, Freedom Plus, and Fortify. **Caution:** There are "hot" oils in this synergy make sure to always dilute.

SPORTS PRO:
Contains - Birch, Peppermint, Nutmeg, Clove, Pennyroyal, Cajeput, Thyme, Black Pepper, Oregano, Marjoram and Cardamom
These oils were selected specifically for their properties that relax, calm, and relieve the tension of spastic muscles resulting from sports injury, fatigue, or stress. It is beneficial for inflammation, assists with broken or bruised bones, sprains, swelling, muscles, and joint discomfort. Sports Pro increases circulation, strengthens the vital centers of the body, and assists in supplying energy during stress, emotional fatigue, and physical weakness.

Sports Pro strengthens the immune system by increasing the white blood cells, supports the adrenals, improves alertness and concentration, benefits the digestive, nervous, and respiratory

systems. It promotes protection, strengthens will power, gives a feeling of courage, bravery, encourages fun, and a zest for life.

Traditional Application: When applied before a workout it will decrease your warm-up time. After a workout rub over all stressed muscles of dilute for a massage. Rub on the back of the neck to relieve stress headaches. Ten drops in the bath helps sore muscles and joints. **Companion Oils:** Peppermint, Basil, Clove Buds, Freedom Plus, True Blue, Pain EZ, Soothing Relief, Nerve Repair, Rejuvenate, Migraine Relief, and Relief.

SUPPORT:
Contains – Organic Clary Sage, Patchouli, and Spikenard
It was formulated to assist the cravings associated with addictive substances. It is relaxing, calms restlessness, strengthens the immune system, assists in recovery from stress related conditions, and improves concentration. In mid-life crisis Support may exert a balancing influence when used in times of personal challenge or change, especially when there is external stress and pressure. Inspires devotion, deep inner peace, assists in finding inner balance in emotional, spiritual, and physical issues. Just smelling this oil is very calming, it diminishes depression, and eases anxiety. Use in conjunction with Rejuvenate.

Traditional Application: Whenever you feel an urge to smoke use two or three drops of Rejuvenate under the tongue and then smelling the Support. It has been reported to be very effective. You may also want to apply at least three drops of Aligning to the bottom of each foot. **Companion Oils:** Love, Confidence, Rejuvenate, Grateful, Angel Assist, Uplifting, Balance, and DNA Repair.

TONING:
Contains – Fennel, Orange, Geranium, Lemongrass, Patchouli, Petitgrain, Spruce, Pine, Cypress, Myrrh, Vetiver, Lavender, and Nutmeg
It is a general tonic restoring muscle tone, increasing cell and tissue healing and regeneration, tightens

and tones the muscles to prevent sagging skin after weight loss. It restores and balances depleted adrenal glands, stimulates the lymphatic system, detoxifies and tones connective tissue and epidermis through capillary stimulation improving cell restorative power.

It assists toning the digestive track, digesting starchy foods and fats, eases inflammation and restores moisture to dry and dehydrated skin. It is beneficial for stretch marks, wrinkles, skin allergies, chapped skin, scaring, integrates energy to all areas of the body balancing the upper and lower chakras, and assists absorption of Vitamin C which strengthens the cellular walls and helps with bruising.

Traditional Application: best applied to warm moist skin after a shower or bath. Always remember to apply over the adrenal areas on the back for better results. **Companion Oils:** Lemon, Tangerine (assists in breaking down cellulite fat pockets), Grapefruit, Mandarin, and Citrus Plus.

TRUE BLUE:
Contains - Wintergreen, Peppermint (India), Blue Tansy, Helichrysum gymnocephalium, German Chamomile, and Spruce
According to modern medicine, more than half the population suffer from inflammation that cause pain and discomfort, and is linked to almost *every* degenerative disease, from heart disease, and diabetes to cancer. The oils hold within them some of the most functional chemical compounds for dealing with inflammation known to man. And, unlike the over-the-counter drugs available on the market today, these compounds are not only effective, they are *safe*.

The oils in True Blue have been synergistically blended to produce what can seem like miraculous results, penetrating deep into the body's tissues to reduce inflammation, ease achy joints and sore muscles, and provide truly amazing relief that lasts. It promotes peace, eases anxiety, is calming, and very soothing.

Traditional Application: apply directly to areas of discomfort. The cool, therapeutic benefits will be felt almost immediately. True Blue can be used with a hot wet compress topically and diffused into the air.
Companion Oils: Lavender, Birch, Clove Buds, Peppermint, Relief, Soothing Relief, Sports Pro, Freedom Plus, and Pain EZ.

TUMMY RUB:
Contains – Peppermint, Juniper Berry, Anise, Fennel, Ginger Root, and Tarragon
It is beneficial in digesting toxic materials, in alleviating indigestion, cramps, upset stomach, vomiting, belching, bloating, heartburn, gas, colic, nervous tension, anxiety, and stress. Tummy Rub is beneficial for spasms, infections, viruses, bacteria, and inflammation. It improves circulation, is toning to the liver, kidneys, spleen, and improves overall body functions. Tummy Rub assists the liver in producing enzymes, balances intestinal activity, relieves discomfort, motion sickness, jet lag, morning sickness, urinary tract infections, diarrhea, and may neutralize negative emotions. It may assist in digesting and assimilate new ideas and has been known to help alleviating parasites (also in animals) by massage and then applying a compress across the stomach.

Traditional Application: apply to the feet and ankles. Massage over the stomach area and apply a hot wet towel compress. When applied on the thymus it may ease gagging reflexes. Applied behind the ears has alleviated morning sickness for some, while others have not experienced these results which goes to show how different we are. For motion sickness apply over the stomach.
Companion Oils: Black Cumin, Fennel, Basil, Tangerine, Peppermint, True Blue, Soothing Relief, Freedom Plus, Relief, and Circle of Life. **Caution:** this may be "hot" for young children and some adults. Be ready to dilute if necessary.

UPLIFTING:
Contains – Ylang Ylang Extra, Cedarwood, Neroli, Melissa, and Jasmine
These oils were combined because of their uplifting

effect as they heal the mind, body, and spirit. It relieves depression, anxiety, and dissolves emotional blocks that may hinder personal growth. Uplifting is soothing to the nervous system, dispelling fear and anger, bringing acceptance, understanding, and assists in dealing with past emotional stress related problems. It clears mental cobwebs and arouses an appreciation for beauty in the world enhancing confidence and self-esteem.

Traditional Application: when there is tension, shock, grief, frustration, and emotional coldness you may experience as instant uplifting calming feeling that comes over you as you breathe in the aroma. Apply to the forehead, temples, ears, wrists, and heart. **Companion Oils**: Love, Utopia, Balance, Grateful, Guardian, Overcome, and Forgiveness.

UTOPIA:
Contains – Valerian Root, Sandalwood, Spruce, Frankincense, Lavender, Helichrysum italicum, Geranium, Petitgrain, and Rose Otto
It was formulated to assists in overcoming traumatic situations, feelings of depression, and anxiety. It balances extremes in emotions, heals emotional wounds, supportive and uplifting in cases of low self-confidence or fear. It assists in overcoming feelings of despair, being pushed over the edge, and letting go of the negative past. Utopia assists in removing negative programming from the cells, increases oxygen around the pineal and pituitary glands. Since the first ingredient is Valerian Root it does have a stinky feet smell but it is very beneficial oil.

Traditional Application: apply to areas of abuse, use in a massage, and add to bath water. To release past or present feelings of abandonment, hurt, fear, and abuse. Sit quietly and breathe in Utopia deeply, blowing out forcefully and let the old emotions release on the out breath. **Companion Oils:** Angel Assist, Confidence, Grateful, Break Thru, Guardian, Love, and Uplifting.

VANILLA BLEND:
Contains – Vanilla and FCO
Beneficial as a nerve sedative, calms emotions, eases tensions, anger, frustration, and brings warm memories. **Traditional Application:** apply on the bottom of the feet, on the shoulders, neck, ears, forehead, over the heart, and liver. **Companion Oils:** Rose, Sandalwood, Orange, Peacemaker, Angel Assist, Love, and Uplifting.

VISION:
Contains – Helichrysum italicum, Frankincense, Lavender, Cypress, Eucalyptus globulus, and Lemongrass
Vision was formulated to strengthen, repair, and improve the eyesight. It improves circulation, fights inflammation, and strengthens blood capillary walls. It is beneficial to fight infection, assist in healing and regenerating connective tissue, is detoxifying, a blood cleanser, and pain reliever. Vision tones muscles and tissue, carries oxygen to the brain, is strengthening and soothing to the nerves, uplifting, and heals emotions. **Remember to avoid putting directly in the eye.**

Traditional Application: lie down, close your eyes, apply on the eyelids, and on the bony part around each eye. Keep your eyes closed and rest a few minutes. Best to use when your eyes can remain closed. Eye problems represent the capacity to see clearly – past, present, and future. It represents fear and a good affirmation is "I see with love and joy." **Companion Oils:** Love, Break Thru, Forgiveness, Balance, and Grateful.

VITALITY:
Contains - Spearmint, Myrtle, Sage, Nutmeg, Geranium, Myrrh, and German Chamomile
It was formulated to support and improve one's own vitality. It assists the respiratory, digestive, and glandular systems. Vitality is beneficial for the lymphatic system, is neuro-balancing, a heart stimulant, relieves depression, inflammation, and improves balance of the thyroid. It is effective for hormonal disturbances and has been known to release emotional blocks related to the past bringing balance. It may alleviate hot flashes and stimulate weight loss by improving metabolic function. Vitality supports the adrenal glands, is a general stimulant

for increasing energy, soothing for anxiety and stress related complaints. It has been reported beneficial when used on location for prostate problems. This oil combination has been recognized for being beneficial for strengthening the complete body. It is known to promote peace, happiness, clarity, adds fun, zest, and enchantment to life.

Traditional Application: Put on thyroid, kidneys, liver (right front), pancreas (left front), and glands. When applied over the throat it may help a person express their true feelings. **Companion Oils:** Fortify, Confidence, Guardian, First Aid, Spice Traders, Geranium, Nutmeg, Lavender, and Frankincense.

~~~~~~~~~~

CARRIER OILS – 100% PURE AND NATURAL

The long shelf life and healing prosperities of Jojoba and Fractionated Coconut Oil (FCO) make them the most beneficial carrier oils to use in your blending. Many carrier oils such as grape seed, almond, or sesame will go rancid within just a few months without any refrigeration. Avoid using rancid oil because that will destroy some of the healing prosperities of the essential oils.

FORAHA, also known as Calophyllum (Madagascar), is used in our Helichrysum & Florah blend. It is considered a carrier oil and is beneficial used for analgesic, sciatica, rheumatism, ulcers, diabetic and atomic wounds, zona lesions, neuritis due to leprosy, physical and chemical burns, radiodermatitis, fissure of post surgical wounds; use as base or additive; caution with sensitive skin since this oil contains irritant properties.

FRACTIONATED COCONUT OIL (F.C.O.) (Malaysia Holland refined): Contents – refined coconut oil consists mainly of saturated fatty acids which is the closest substance to human sub-cutaneous fat and more compatible with skin than vegetable oils; a very clean with no irritants and does not go rancid. Massage therapists like this oil because it does not stain sheets.

JOJOBA (USA): Contents – protein, minerals, plant wax, myristic acid, mimics sebum. It assists eczema, psoriasis, hair care, and all skin types.

~~~~~~~~~~

BLENDING ESSENTIAL OILS:

When making your own blends here is what I use. Six drops of essential oil to ¼ oz carrier oil; 12 to 15 drops of essential oil to ½ oz carrier oil, and 24 to 30 drops of essential oil to one ounce of carrier oil.

For a child or a sick person use only half the amount of drops mentioned. On an infant use only a drop of essential oil to ¼ ounce of carrier oil. The essential oils are very concentrated. Even using them in such small amounts you will see the benefits without causing a detoxifying effect on your little clients.

ALPHABETICAL LISTING

IMPORTANT: This information is for educational purposes only. It is not provided in order to diagnose, prescribe or treat any disease, illness or injured condition of the body. Its intention is solely informational and educational. Anyone suffering from any disease, illness or injury should consult with a health care professional.

Essential oils work well for emotional and physical ailments. For each application listed below, you will find several choices of oils that may be used. Some suggested ways to use the oils would be:

- To smell the aroma by breathing in deeply and exhale forcefully
- Apply a drop of the oil to each ear and massage in gently
- Rub a few drops on the bottom of the feet and massage
- Massage gently across the forehead and temples
- Use 6 to 10 drops in carrier oil for a full body massage
- Add 6 to 8 drops to your bath water

When you first begin using the oils, it is best to only use three or four at a time diluted in carrier oil. It is important to know how quickly oils can deal with your emotions. When you understand that smell is the quickest way to release an emotion, it will not surprise you if when applying the essential oils you feel like crying. This happens once in a while and is all right. Just breathe deeply and blow out forcefully several times to release the emotion that is coming up.

Avoid getting caught up in analyzing the emotion. Let it go and be done with. Just breathe, cry and blow. Feel the energy of the emotion being wrapped with love and peace. Breathe and blow until you feel the peace within. The Confidence essential oil is a good one to apply to bring you back into balance. The Emotional Workbook and Training Kit explain the benefits of using the oils for emotional release. Louise Hay's book, Heal Thy Self, explains how emotions actually cause our physical health problems.

It has been shown that adding minerals, enzymes, probiotics, Nature's Nutrients, Ageless Plus, whole raw foods and sprouts to your diet along with using the essential oils has been beneficial in assisting the body with important building blocks to overcoming disease.

Because of the chemical constituents such as aldehydes, azulene, carvacrol, esters, phenols, and sesquiterpenes in the oils, they may be beneficial for the applications listed below. The oils are very versatile and, as you use them, you will find some you really like for certain conditions. **Remember** this section of the book is only suggested ways of using the Essential Oils. Underline the ones you like to use or, if the oil is not on the list under a specific topic just add it to the list so you will have a quick reference. This is your workbook to use and enjoy.

IMPORTANT: After each symptom you will find a list of oils. They are not listed in any specific order of effectiveness. After you read the list refer to the Single and Blends Sections of the Workbook for more specific information on the oil. This way you are able to choose the one best suited for your needs.

ALPHABETICAL LISTINGS

Abscess: Tea Tree, Thyme, Gentle Healer, Fortify

Absent Minded: Basil, Rosemary, Peppermint, Focus, Brain Power

Abuse: Geranium, Lavender, Angel Assist, Confidence, Break Thru, Utopia, Balance, Love

Acceptance: Confidence, DNA Repair, Awareness, Hope, Love, Uplifting

Aches & Pains: Birch, Basil, Soothing Relief, True Blue, Relief, Sports Pro, Pain EZ

Acid pH: When you first wake up, drink a glass of warm water with several drops of the lemon oil. Eat foods that contain the alkaline minerals of calcium, molybdenum, magnesium, and potassium. Use pH Balance.

Acne: Cucumber, Lavender, Baby Soft, Freedom, and Skin Care.

ADD: Grounding, Serenity, Vetiver

Addictions: Bergamot, Purify, Serenity, Support, Rejuvenate – Using Balance along the jaw has been beneficial.

Adrenal Cortex: Nutmeg, Sage, Geranium, Pine Needles, Spruce, Vitality, Toning

Aging: Rosewood, Frankincense, Cucumber, Geranium, Myrrh, Sandalwood, Elemi, Rose, Baby Soft, Freedom, Skin Care

AIDS: Helichrysum, Black Cumin, Exodus, Fortify, Spice Traders, Ageless

Air Pollution: Lemon, Lavender, Spice Traders, Rosemary, Eucalyptus, Resp EZ, Purify, Joyful

Alcoholism: Angelica Root, Fennel, Ginger, Serenity, Rejuvenate, Circle of Life, Purify

Alertness: Basil, Peppermint, Rosemary, Lemon, Citrus Plus, Focus

Alkalizing: Black Cumin, Lavender, Lemon, Lime, Mandarin, Citrus Plus, Tangerine, Tarragon, Valerian Root, Wintergreen

Allergies: Eucalyptus, Lavender, Resp EZ, Spice Traders, Fortify, Breathe EZ

Alopecia: Rosemary

Alzheimer's: Cedarwood, Frankincense, Sandalwood, Rosemary, Cypress, Focus, Grounding, Peppermint

Ambition: Rosemary, Faith, Passion for Life, Focus, Magnify, Balance, Grateful, Prosperity

Amenorrhea (lack of menstruation): Basil, Carrot Seed, Fennel, Hyssop, Juniper Berry, Marjoram, Myrrh, Rose, Hormone Balance

Amoebic Dysentery: Clove, Fortify

Analgesic: Clove, Rosemary

Anemia: Lemon, Rosemary, Fortify, Exodus, Freedom Plus

Anesthesia: Helichrysum, Clove Bud, Relief, Soothing Relief, True Blue, Sport Pro

Aneurysm: Frankincense, Helichrysum, Cypress, Circle of Life

Anger: Lavender, Frankincense, Sandalwood, Break Thru, Serenity, Confidence, Mountain Retreat, Calming, Balance, Peaceful Moments

Angina: Orange (false angina), Pain EZ, True Blue, Soothing Relief, Relief, Sport Pro

53

Anorexia: Tarragon, Calming, Grapefruit, Joyous, Citrus Plus

Anthrax: Rose, Thyme

Anti-Coagulant: Helichrysum, Tangerine

Anti-Depressant: Break Thru, Hope, Citrus Plus, Balance, Frankincense, Lavender, Geranium, Rosewood, Orange, DNA Repair

Anti-Inflammatory: Basil. Clove, Helichrysum, Spruce, Gentle Healer, Relief, Soothing Relief, True Blue, Sports Pro, Fortify, Nerve Repair

Anti-Microbial: Black Cumin, Cinnamon Bark, Palmarosa, Thyme, Fortify, Prosperity, Exodus, Spice Traders, Rejuvenate

Anti-Oxidant: Cedarwood, Frankincense, Exodus, Spice Traders, Fortify, Purify

Anti-Spasmodic: Basil, Black Cumin, Clove Bud, Marjoram, Peppermint, Birch, Spruce, Relief, Pain EZ, Sport Pro, Nerve Repair

Antiseptic: Basil, Clove, Lemon, Oregano, Peppermint, Tea Tree, Thyme, Nerve Repair, Spice Traders, Purify, Fortify, Citrus Plus

Anti-Viral: Black Cumin, Cinnamon Bark, Clove, Hyssop, Melissa, Mountain Savory, Oregano, Ravintsara, Exodus, Spice Traders

Anxiety: Frankincense, Geranium, Balance, Joyful, Confidence, Serenity, Hope, Lavender Mountain Retreat, Peaceful Moments

Apathy: Peaceful Moments, Jasmine, Orange, Geranium, Peppermint, Rosemary, Rosewood, Sandalwood, Confidence, Calming

Aphrodisiac: Ylang Ylang, Neroli, Jasmine, Patchouli, Sandalwood

Appetite--Loss of: Bergamot, Ginger, Nutmeg, Lime, Balance, Confidence

Apnea (Asphyxia - breathing stops temporarily)**:** Peppermint, Confidence, Focus, Rosemary

Arterial Hypertension: Ylang Ylang, Cypress, Circle of Life, Black Cumin

Arterial Vasodilator: Marjoram, Cypress, Circle of Life, Vitality, Freedom Plus

Arteries: Lavender, Cypress, Ginger, Gentle Healer, Circle of Life

Arthritis: Soothing Relief, True Blue, Relief, Helichrysum, Clove Buds, Sports Pro, Pain EZ, Freedom Plus,

Asthma: Resp EZ, Breathe EZ, Basil, Clove, Cypress, Eucalyptus, Frankincense, Tea Tree, Hyssop, Marjoram, Melissa, Black Cumin, Fortify, Peppermint, Rosemary, Spice Traders

Astringent: Cypress, Geranium, Lemon, Sage, Helichrysum, Cucumber

Athlete's Foot: Black Cumin, Clove, Lavender, Patchouli, Myrrh, Eucalyptus, Lemon, Tea Tree, Freedom Plus, Gentle Healer, Fortify

Attitude: Citrus Plus, Calming, Confidence, Mountain Retreat, Love, Hormone Balance, Uplifting, Magnify, Serenity, Balance, Faith

Attraction: DNA Repair, Love, Confidence, Prosperity, Balance, Peaceful Moments

Autoimmune: Black Cumin, Frankincense, Oregano, Mountain Savory, Exodus, Fortify, Spice Traders, Freedom Plus

Autistic Children: Vetiver, Grounding

Awareness: Lemon, Focus, Envision, Magnify

Baby: Neroli, Rose, Angel, Baby Soft, Love, DNA Repair – always dilute for babies – 3-5 drops oil with 1/4 ounce of carrier oil.

Back: Soothing Relief, Relief, True Blue, Confidence, Basil, Marjoram, Eucalyptus, Ginger, Nerve Repair, Sports Pro, Freedom Plus

Bacteria: Cinnamon Bark, Oregano, Clove, Peppermint, Ravintsara, Rosemary, Fortify, Spice Traders, Rejuvenate, Freedom Plus

Balance: Cedarwood, Frankincense, Ylang Ylang, Sandalwood, Confidence, Balance, Mountain Retreat, Grateful, Citrus Plus

Baldness: Cedarwood, Rosemary, Juniper Berry, Sandalwood, Ylang Ylang, Holy Basil, Hair Support, Cucumber

Behavior Modification: Serenity, Faith, Love, Grounding, DNA Repair, Faith

Bell's palsy: Freedom, Nerve Repair

Bladder: Lemongrass, Juniper Berry, Gentle Healer, Vitality, Rejuvenate, Freedom Plus

Bleeding: Cypress, Geranium, Lemon, Circle of Life, Helichrysum

Blemishes: Frankincense, Rose, Freedom, Circle of Life, Freedom Plus, Skin Care

Blister: Lavender, Chamomile, Eucalyptus, Lemon, Helichrysum, Tea Tree, Gentle Healer

Blood: Lemon, Helichrysum, Fredom, Circle of Life, Exodus, Spice Traders, Fortify

Blood Pressure: Lavender, Lemon (lowers), Marjoram, Freedom (lowers), Ylang Ylang (lowers), Rosemary (raises), Thyme (raises), Circle of Life, Serenity, Freedom Plus

Blood Vessels: Geranium, Marjoram, Circle of Life, Freedom Plus, Freedom, Cypress

Boils: Bergamot, Lavender, Lemon, Juniper, Helichrysum, Fortify, Exodus, Spice Traders

Bones: Birch, Spruce, Ginger, Juniper Berry, Peppermint, Sandalwood, Relief, Sport Pro

Bowels: Ginger, Peppermint, Anise Seed, Black Cumin, Fennel, Freedom Plus, Tummy Rub

Brain: Clary Sage, Helichrysum, Geranium, Cypress, Peppermint, Rosemary, Spearmint, Frankincense, Sandalwood, Nerve Repair, Focus, Brain Power, Grounding

Breast: Cypress, Geranium, Lemongrass, Jasmine, Clary Sage, Fennel (firms), Baby Soft, Toning, Skin Care

Brittle Nails: Lemon, Freedom

Bronchitis: Basil, Black Cumin, Clove, Fir, Cypress, Eucalyptus, Frankincense, Hyssop, Melissa, Myrtle, Oregano, Rosemary, Exodus, Freedom Plus, Fortify, Breathe EZ, Spice Traders

Bruises: Gentle Healer, Relief, Freedom Plus, Lavender, Marjoram, Sport Pro, Nerve Repair

Bulimia: Grapefruit, Break Thru, Serenity, Joyous, Balance, Confidence

Bunions: Chamomile, Lemon, Ravintsara, Birch, Eucalyptus, Soothing Relief

Burns: Lavender, Chamomile, Clove Bud, Geranium, Tea Tree, Ravintsara, Helichrysum, Gentle Healer, Freedom

Bursitis: Birch, Basil, Marjoram, Spruce, Relief, Pain EZ, Soothing Relief, True Blue, Sport Pro, Mountain Retreat

Calcification of bones: Relief, Sports Pro, Soothing Relief, True Blue

Calming: Lavender, Orange, Tangerine, Ylang Ylang, Angel Assist, Citrus Plus, Serenity, Calming, Peaceful Moments

Cancer: Frankincense, Clove Bud, Oregano, Lemon, Exodus, Fortify, Lemongrass, Love, Spice Traders, Joyful

Candida: Bergamot (vaginal), Geranium, Clary Sage, Tea Tree, Oregano, Patchouli, Rosemary, Rosewood, Tummy Rub, Freedom Plus, Fortify (Candida lives in the acid condition in the body).

Cankers: Lavender, Myrrh, Melaleuca, Tea Tree, Freedom Plus, Fortify

Cardiac Insufficiency: Circle of Life, Rose Blend, Helichrysum

Cardiac Spasm: Rose, Orange, Petitgrain, Marjoram, Sport Pro, Circle of Life

Cardiovascular System: See Heart

Carpal Tunnel: Spruce, Peppermint, Birch, Marjoram, Helichrysum, Relief, Sports Pro, Freedom Plus, Nerve Repair, True Blue, Soothing Relief

Cataracts: Lavender, Cypress, Frankincense, Lemongrass, Vision

Catarrh: Cedarwood, Frankincense, Hyssop, Lavender, Lemon, Myrtle, Rosemary, Tea Tree, Breathe EZ, Spice Traders, Fortify, Purify

Cavities: Spice Traders, Tea Tree

Cells: Nerve Repair, Lemon, All Around, Toning, Rejuvenate

Cellulite: Grapefruit, Juniper Berry, Rosemary, Tangerine, Slim and Trim, Birch, Cypress, Lemon, Geranium, Fennel, Thyme, Toning

Cerebro-spinal meningitis: Oregano, Exodus, Fortify, Spice Traders, Helichrysum

Change: Lavender, Angel Assist, Balance, Grounding, Break Thru, Faith, In The Moment, DNA Repair, Magnify, Serenity

Chemical Detoxification: Rejuvenate, MSM

Chickenpox: Bergamot, Chamomile, Eucalyptus, Lavender, Tea Tree, Freedom, Helichrysum (scars)

Childbirth: Clary Sage, Angel Assist, Baby Soft, Rose, Jasmine, Confidence

Childhood Diseases: Lavender, Myrtle, Freedom Plus, Spice Traders, Exodus, Fortify

Chills: Peppermint, Black Cumin, Grapefruit, Freedom Plus, Ginger (6 drops in hot bath)

Cholera: Clove Bud, Ravintsara, Rosemary, Exodus, Spice Traders, Fortify

Cholesterol: Clary Sage, Rosemary, Helichrysum

Chronic Fatigue: Lavender, Peppermint, Oregano, Melaleuca, Nutmeg, Exodus, Spice Traders, Freedom Plus, Fortify, Focus

Circulation: Birch, Basil, Cypress, Hyssop, Peppermint, Rosemary, Eucalyptus, Ginger, Lemon, Juniper Berry, Nutmeg, Circle of Life, Freedom Plus, Focus, First Aid. Toning, Flu-Time

Cirrhosis of the Liver: Break Thru, Lemon

Clarity: Basil, Peppermint, Rosemary, Spearmint, Focus

Claustrophobia: Clary Sage, Confidence, Serenity, Citrus Plus, Calming

Cleanser: Tea Tree, Rosemary, Tummy Rub, Lemon, Break Thru, Citrus Plus, Purify

Colds: Basil, Clove Bud, Eucalyptus, Fir, Frankincense, Ginger, Grapefruit, Tea Tree, Hyssop, Lemon, Myrtle, Oregano, Peppermint, Rosemary, Thyme, Breathe EZ, Exodus, Spice Traders, Fortify

Cold Sores: Bergamot, Lavender, Tea Tree, Freedom, Gentle Healer

Colic: Chamomile, Ginger, Lavender, Marjoram, Peppermint, Rosemary, Tummy Rub

Colitis: Clove Bud, Rosemary, Tarragon, Thyme, Tummy Rub

Coma: Frankincense, Sandalwood, Myrrh, Confidence, Balance, Focus

Compassion: Rose, Geranium, Angel Assist, Confidence, Peaceful Moments, Love, Balance, Citrus Plus, Faith

Complexion: Cucumber, Lavender, Baby Soft, Passion for Life, Freedom, Skin Care

Concentration: Basil, Lemon, Patchouli, Peppermint, Rosemary, Focus

Confidence: Spruce, Frankincense, Myrtle, Confidence, Magnify, Guardian, Faith

Confusion: Basil, Cedarwood, Cypress, Fir, Frankincense, Peppermint, Spruce, Focusing, Balance, Aligning, Mind-Alive, Gratitude

Congestion: Cedarwood, Eucalyptus, Fir, Ginger, Hyssop, Peppermint, Pine, Ravintsara, Rosemary, Breathe EZ, Exodus, Spice Traders, Fortify, Resp EZ

Consciousness: Lavender, Lemon, Peppermint, Rosemary, Basil, Focusing, Frankincense, Sandalwood

Consoling: Rose, Geranium, Angel Assist, Baby Soft, Love, Mountain Retreat, Peaceful Moments, Serenity, Confidence, Peacemaker

Constipation: Ginger, Fennel, Marjoram, Nutmeg, Palmarosa, Freedom Plus, Tummy Rub

Contagious Disease: Clove Bud, Cinnamon, Ginger, Juniper Berry, Oregano, Thyme, Fortify, Spice Traders

Coronary Blood Vessel Disease: Spice Traders, Rejuvenate, Circle of Life, Freedom Plus, Fortify

Corns: Lemon, Peppermint, Chamomile

Cortisone: Spruce, Birch, Wintergreen

Coughs: Hyssop, Eucalyptus, Fir, Rosemary, Pine, Ravintsara, Cedarwood, Ginger, Juniper Berry, Marjoram, Tea Tree, Myrtle (smokers), Oregano, Breathe EZ, Spice Traders

Chronic Coughs: Melissa, Cypress, Hyssop, Frankincense, Peppermint, Myrrh, Tea Tree

Courage: Clove Bud, Ginger, Black Pepper, Petitgrain Bigarade, Angel Assist, Confidence, Balance, Grounding

Cramps: Basil, Rosemary, Ginger, Peppermint, Marjoram, Sports Pro, Tummy Rub, True Blue, Soothing Relief, Pain EZ, Nerve Repair, Freedom Plus

Creativity: Helichrysum, Jasmine, Orange, Magnify, Citrus Plus, Love, Guardian

Crohn's Disease: Rejuvenate, Freedom Plus, Confidence

Cuts: Clove Bud, Helichrysum, Lavender, Tea Tree, Ravintsara, Gentle Healer, Fortify

Cystic Fibrosis: Black Cumin, Ravintsara

Cystitis: Bergamot, Cedarwood, Chamomile, Eucalyptus, Frankincense, Juniper Berry, Tea Tree, Lavender, Pine, Sandalwood, Fennel, Thyme, Birch, Clove Bud, Freedom Plus

Dandruff: Cedarwood, Holy Basil, Lavender, Patchouli, Rosemary, Sandalwood, Eucalyptus, Lemon, Tea Tree, Freedom Plus, Hair Support

Deafness: Helichrysum italicum (if nerves)

Debility/Poor Muscle Tone: Clary Sage, Lemon, Ginger, Grapefruit, Marjoram, Pine, Rosemary, Petitgrain, Skin Tone, Slim & Trim, Sports Pro

Decongestant: Hyssop, Myrtle, Eucalyptus, Rosemary, Breathe EZ, Spice Traders

Degenerative Joint Disease: Rejuvenate, Relief, True Blue, Soothing Relief, Freedom Plus, Fortify, Sports Pro

Denial: Blend of Rose, Angel Assist, Magnify, Balance, Confidence

Dental Infections: Clove Bud, Myrrh, Tea Tree, Freedom Plus, Fortify, Spice Traders

Deodorizer: Lemon, Citrus Plus, Myrtle, Rosemary, Purify

Depression: Frankincense, Neroli, Geranium, Grapefruit, Jasmine, Lavender, Orange, Rose, Rosewood, Sandalwood, Ylang Ylang, Angel Assist, Balance, Serenity, Citrus Plus, Love, Confidence, Peaceful Moments, Grateful

Dermatitis: Black Cumin, Cedarwood, Cucumber, Chamomile, Geranium, Helichrysum, Lavender, Patchouli, Palmarosa, Rosemary, Baby Soft, Freedom Plus

Detoxifies: Black Cumin, Grapefruit, Juniper Berry, Fennel, Helichrysum, Rosemary, Patchouli (digests toxic material), Fortify, Exodus

Diabetes: Cassia, Eucalyptus, Fennel, Holy Basil, Geranium, Rosemary, Ylang Ylang, Dill, Coriander, Confidence, Freedom Plus, Fortify

Diaper Rash: Lavender, Jasmine, Chamomile, Baby Soft, Freedom Plus, Skin Care, Renew

Diarrhea: Chamomile, Cypress, Ginger, Tea Tree, Myrrh, Nutmeg, Orange, Peppermint, Tangerine, Thyme, Tummy Rub, All Around

Digestion: Anise, Fennel, Ginger, Grapefruit, Lemongrass, Tea Tree, Nutmeg, Tangerine, Peppermint, Pepper, Marjoram (stimulant), Freedom Plus, Circle of Life, Tummy Rub

Diphtheria: Black Cumin

Disc: See Ligaments

Disinfectant: Purify, Gentle Healer, Fortify, Lemon, Citronella, Spice Trader

Disorientation: Rosemary, Peppermint, Love, Focus, Mountain Retreat, Balance, Serenity, Calming, Peaceful Moments

Diuretic: Tangerine, Cypress, Cedarwood, Fennel, Juniper Berry, Orange, Patchouli, Sage, Vitality, Citrus Plus

Dizziness: Tangerine, Peppermint, Frankincense, Sandalwood, Focus

DNA Repair: Cedarwood, Sandalwood, Vetiver, Myrrh, Ginger, Hyssop, Frankincense, Spruce, Peppermint, DNA Repair, Exodus

Down's syndrome: Frankincense, Sandalwood, Focus, Confidence

Drug Withdrawal: Balance, Grapefruit, Fennel, Serenity, Circle of Life, Rejuvenate, Support

Dysentery: Myrrh, Black Cumin, Lemon, Peppermint, Freedom Plus, Tummy Rub

Dyspepsia: Basil, Black Cumin, Grapefruit, Lavender, Lemon, Tummy Rub, Freedom Plus

E. coli: Black Cumin, Exodus, Spice Trader

Earache: The following copals should be diluted with massage oil before putting on a piece of cotton and placing it in the ear: Basil, Lavender, Chamomile, Helichrysum, Fortify, Sandalwood, Gentle Healer, Freedom Plus, Purify, True Blue

Eczema: Chamomile, Geranium, Juniper Berry, Lavender, Myrrh, Patchouli, Cedarwood, Skin Care, Freedom Plus, Cucumber, Renew

Edema: Cypress, Geranium, Juniper Berry, Lemongrass, Orange, Tangerine, Citrus Plus

Elevating: Rose, Petitgrain Bigarade, Angel Assist, Peaceful Moments, Magnify, Love, Faith, Neroli Blend

Emotions: Rose, Cypress, Jasmine (blocks), Lemon (clarity), Myrrh (coldness), Bergamot (wounds), Frankincense (wounds), Ylang Ylang, Sandalwood (clears negative programming from cells), Angel Assist, Mountain Retreat, Love, Joyous, Faith, DNA Repair, Serenity, Balance, Guardian, Peacemaker, Grateful, Euphoria

Emphysema: Basil, Spice Traders, Exodus, Balance, Breathe EZ, Fortify, Resp EZ, Calming

Endocrine System: Cinnamon, Bergamot, Black Pepper, Rosemary, Hormone Balance, Vitality, Confidence, Balance

Endometriosis: Clary Sage, Sage, Geranium, Nutmeg, Fortify, Spice Trader, Gentle Healer

Energy: Cypress, Eucalyptus, Frankincense, Ginger, Rosemary, Balance, Love, Focus, Confidence, Prosperity, Vitality, Magnify

Engorgement of Breasts: Geranium, Black Cumin, Freedom Plus, Vitality, Fortify

Epidemics: Eucalyptus, Oregano, Fortify, Exodus, Spice Trader, Freedom Plus

Epstein Bar Virus: Black Cumin, Mountain Savory, Oregano, Rejuvenate, Spice Traders, Exodus, Fortify

Equilibrium: Ylang Ylang, Peppermint, Focus, Confidence, Balance

Estrogen: Sage, Clary Sage, Anise Seed (estrogen like properties), Hormone Balance

Euphoria: Clary Sage, Jasmine, Peaceful Moments, Calming, Citrus Plus, Love, Passion for Life, Peacemaker

Exhaustion: Peppermint, Black Pepper, Confidence, Serenity, Focus, Calming

Expectorant: Marjoram, Myrrh, Ravintsara, Oregano, Purify, Breathe EZ, Spice Trader, Freedom Plus, Fortify

Excessive Perspiration: Citronella, Cypress, Lemongrass, Petitgrain, Pine Needles, Sage

Eyes: Lemongrass, Cypress, Eucalyptus, Rosewood (pink eye), Vision. **Never put oils in the eyes!**

Fainting: Basil, Lavender, Peppermint, Rosemary, Focus

Fat: Grapefruit, Cypress, Tangerine, Toning,

Slim & Trim, Calming

Fatigue: Clove, Ginger, Peppermint, Nutmeg, Lime, Thyme, Basil (mental), Focus, Calming, Freedom Plus, Confidence, Peaceful Moments

Fear: Rose, Geranium, Myrrh, Sandalwood, Lavender, Angel Assist, Faith, Magnify, Citrus Plus, Love, Break Thru, Mountain Retreat, Serenity, Calming

Feelings: Angel Assist, Break Thru, Calming, Uplifting, Balance, Confidence, In The Moment, Magnify, Mountain Retreat, Peaceful Moments

Fermentation: See Flatulence

Fertility: Frankincense, Geranium, Hormone Balance, Grateful, Confidence, Citrus Plus, Love, Uplifting, Peaceful Moments

Fever: Basil, Peppermint, Cajeput (cholera), Fir, Ginger, Frankincense, Helichrysum, Juniper Berry, Rosemary, Freedom Plus, Gentle Healer

Fibromyalgia: Geranium, Relief, Sport Pro, Fortify, True Blue, Soothing Relief, Freedom Plus.

Flatulence: Tummy Rub, Basil, Ginger, Clove, Fennel, Peppermint, Tarragon

Fleas & Insects: Peppermint, Cedarwood, Tea Tree, Citronella, Purify, Bug Off

Flu: Ginger, Myrtle, Oregano, Peppermint, Ravintsara, Tea Tree, Rosemary, Exodus, Fortify, Freedom Plus, Breathe EZ, Resp EZ, Spice Traders, First Aid

Fluid Retention: Cypress, Grapefruit, Lavender, Rosemary, Tangerine, Orange, Citrus Plus

Food Poisoning: Tummy Rub, Juniper Berry, Freedom Plus, Fortify

Forgiveness: Rose, Angel Assist, Balance, Love, Grateful, Uplifting

Fortifying: Mountain Retreat, Spice Traders, Fortify, Rejuvenate, Exodus, Confidence

Freckles: Helichrysum, Frankincense, Skin Care, Renew

Frigidity: Clary Sage, Jasmine, Neroli, Nutmeg, Sandalwood, Rosewood, Ylang Ylang

Frustration: Ylang Ylang, Angel Assist, Joyous, Confidence, Magnify, Citrus Plus, Balance, Love, Guardian, Serenity

Fungus: Melaleuca, Mountain Savory, Oregano, Ravintsara, Thyme, Gentle Healer, Exodus, Freedom Plus, Spice Traders, Fortify

Gallbladder: Geranium, Helichrysum

Gallstones: Lemon, Peppermint

Gas: See Flatulence

Gastritis: Sandalwood, Sage, Peppermint, Ginger, Tummy Rub, Freedom Plus

Generosity: Orange, Love, Balance, Citrus Plus, Grateful, Peaceful Moments

Genitals: Clary Sage

Gentleness: Rose, Rosewood, Angel Assist, Love, Focus, Balance, Peacemaker, Baby Soft, Passion for Life, Confidence, Uplifting

Gingivitis: Myrrh, Tea Tree, Freedom Plus, Fortify, Spice Traders (brush teeth)

Glandular System: Sage, Spearmint, Spruce, Vitality, Hormone Balance, Rejuvenate

Glucose: Cinnamon Bark, Cassia

Gonorrhea: Black Cumin, Sandalwood, Freedom Plus, Rejuvenate, Fortify

Gout: Basil, Hyssop, Nutmeg, Rosemary, Juniper Berry, Thyme, Relief, Soothing Relief, True Blue, Sport Pro

Gratitude: Orange, Rose, Angel Assist, Utopia, Balance, Grateful, Uplifting, Peacemaker, Citrus Plus, Love, Peaceful Moments, Mountain Retreat

Grief: Rose (Two drops rubbed over the heart), Tangerine, Love, Aligning, Angel, Blossoms, Balance, Tranquility, Citrus Passion, Mind-Alive

Griping Pains: Fennel, Peppermint, Tummy Rub, Soothing Relief, Relief, True Blue

Grounding: Fir, Lavender, Spruce, Hormone Balance, Confidence, Balance, Grounding

Grudges: Lemon, Orange, DNA Repair, Love, Balance, Confidence, Citrus Plus, Magnify, Serenity, Grateful, Peaceful Moments

Gum Disease: Tea Tree, Gentle Healer, Freedom Plus, Spice Traders (brush teeth)

Hair: Basil, Clary Sage, Grapefruit, Lavender, Sage, Cedarwood, Cypress, Hair Support

Halitosis: Bergamot, Fennel, Lavender, Myrrh, Nutmeg, Peppermint, Fortify, Spice Traders

Hangovers: Fennel, Grapefruit, Lavender, Lemon, Rosemary, Focus, Freedom Plus

Happiness: Rose, Joyous, Focus, Balance, Love, Mountain Retreat, Confidence, Angel Assist, Citrus Plus, Peaceful Moments

Hay Fever: Black Cumin, Breathe EZ, Spice Traders, Confidence, Balance, Fortify

Headache: Peppermint, Helichrysum, Lavender, Thyme, Relief, True Blue, Soothing Relief, Freedom Plus, Migraine Relief, Sport Pro, Focus

Healing: Helichrysum, Clove Bud, Cypress, Eucalyptus, Lemon, Sandalwood, Gentle Healer, Citrus Plus, Balance, Love, Calming

Health: Black Cumin, Lemon, Lavender, Tea Tree, Oregano, Ravintsara, Rosemary, Fortify, Freedom Plus, Exodus, Rejuvenate, Spice Traders, First Aid, Toning, Slim and Trim, Confidence, Uplifting, True Blue

Hearing Problems: Helichrysum Italicum (if nerves), Nerve Repair, DNA Repair

Heart: Rose, Ylang Ylang, Orange, Angel Assist, Circle of Life, Hormone Balance, Citrus Plus, Peaceful Moments, Confidence, Love, Grateful, Balance

Heartburn: Black Pepper, Chamomile, Lemon, Peppermint, Tummy Rub, Freedom Plus, Soothing Relief

Heat: Peppermint in water, Relieve the Heat

Hematoma: Helichrysum, Circle of Life

Hemorrhaging: Helichrysum, Rose, Lemon

Hemorrhoids: Cypress, Myrtle, Soothing Relief, Circle of Life, Freedom Plus, Vitality

Hepatitis C: Fortify, Rejuvenate, Spice Traders, Exodus

Hernias: Basil, Cypress, Helichrysum, Ginger, Geranium, Lavender, Rosemary, Relieve Me, Soothing Relief, All Around, Tummy Rub

Herpes: Black Cumin, Eucalyptus, Lavender, Lemon, Tea Tree, Ravintsara, Freedom Plus, Exodus, Fortify, Spice Traders

Hiccups: Coriander, Fennel, Tarragon, Sandalwood, Tummy Rub

High Blood Pressure: Lemon, Black Cumin, Ylang Ylang, Melissa, Lavender, Marjoram, Clary Sage, Freedom Plus, Circle of Life

Hives: Patchouli, Chamomile, Baby Skin, Freedom, Vitamin C Plus

Hoarseness: Jasmine, Myrrh, Balance, Spice Traders, Break Thru, Citrus Plus

Hodgkin's Disease: Clove Bud, Frankincense, Joyous, Soothing Relief, Sport Pro, Relief, Freedom Plus

Hormone: Clary Sage, Geranium, Myrtle, Spearmint, Spikenard (regulates), Bergamot, Rose, Circle of Life, Hormone Balance

Hostility: Clary Sage, Confidence, Angel Assist, Rose, Love, Balance, Peacemaker, Citrus Plus, Uplifting, Magnify, Peaceful Moments, Calming

Hot Flashes: Peppermint, Clary Sage, Bergamot, Vitality, Hormone Balance

Hurt (emotional): Geranium, Rose, Lavender, Angel, Balance, Tranquility, Aligning, Love, Trauma-Gone, Guardian, Mind-Alive, Uplift

Hyper-Thyroidism: Myrrh, Myrtle, Vitality

Hyperactivity: Clary Sage, Vetiver, Calming, Serenity, Citrus Plus, Confidence, Support

Hyperpnoea: Ylang Ylang, Resp EZ, Breathe EZ, Spice Traders

Hypertension: Spearmint, Clove Bud, Marjoram, Confidence, Balance, Freedom Plus

Hypo-Cholesterol: Helichrysum

Hypoglycemia: Eucalyptus, Black Cumin, Geranium, Cinnamon Bark, Fortify, Freedom

Hysteria: Lavender, Serenity, Confidence, Balance, Peaceful Moments, Citrus Plus, Tea Tree, Calming

Immune Function: Frankincense, Black Cumin, Cinnamon Bark, Lemon, Mountain Savory, Clove Thyme, Rosemary, Oregano, Fortify, Exodus, Freedom Plus, Prosperity, Spice Traders

Impetigo: Black Cumin, Patchouli, Tea Tree, Gentle Healer, Spice Traders

Impotence: Clove, Ginger, Clary Sage, Nutmeg, Sandalwood, Rose, Ylang Ylang, Vitality

Indigestion: Tummy Rub, Black Cumin, Ginger, Peppermint, Fennel, Marjoram, Nutmeg, Thyme, Rosemary, Freedom Plus, Soothing Relief

Infection: Cinnamon Bark, Lavender, Oregano, Tea Tree, Ravintsara, Rosemary, Clove Bud, Lemon, Frankincense, Freedom Plus, Exodus, Spice Traders, Gentle Healer, Fortify

Infertility: Clary Sage, Geranium, Lymph Detox

Inflammation: Helichrysum, Chamomile, Lavender, Birch, Eucalyptus, Frankincense, Hyssop, Peppermint, Spruce, Relieve Me, Sport Pro, All Around, Fortify, Immune Strength, First Aid, True Blue, Soothing Relief, Migraine Relief

Inner Child: Lavender, Angel Assist, Love, Uplifting, Balance, Peacemaker, DNA Repair

Insect Bites: Lavender, Basil, Eucalyptus, Patchouli, Thyme, Chamomile, Tea Tree, Purify, Gentle Healer, Freedom, Bug Free

Insect Repellent: Bug Off, Basil, Clove, Eucalyptus, Lemongrass, Citronella, Tea Tree, Rosemary, Peppermint, Freedom, Bug Free

Insecticide: Patchouli, Purify, Tea Tree

Insecurity: Frankincense, Lavender, Angel Assist, Confidence, Mountain Retreat, Calming, Balance, Grounding, Citrus Plus, Peaceful Moments

Insomnia: Chamomile, Lavender, Valerian, Ylang Ylang, Serenity, Citrus Plus, Calming, Peaceful Moments

Insulin: Holy Basil, Coriander, Dill, Vitality

Intelligence: Patchouli, Basil (fatigue), Peppermint, Focusing, Brainstorm

Intestines: Tarragon (sluggish & spasm), Clove Bud (parasites), Lemon (parasites), Fennel (parasites & spasm), Basil (parasites), Marjoram (peristalsis), Tangerine (spasm), Freedom (worms), Tummy Rub

Intuition: Jasmine, Rose, Focus, Balance, Angel Assist, DNA Repair, Guardian, Dreamtime, Love, Magnify, Grateful, Joyous, Meditation

Irritability: Myrrh, Rose, Love, Confidence, Citrus Plus, Hormone Balance, Balance, Magnify, Mountain Retreat, Serenity, Calming

Itchy Skin: Lavender, Cucumber, Cedarwood, Juniper, Myrrh, Patchouli, Tea Tree, Skin Care, Rosewood, Chamomile, Baby Soft, Freedom

Jet Lag: Peppermint, Rosewood, Confidence, Balance, Serenity, Love, Fortify, Freedom Plus

Jock Itch: Tea Tree, Myrrh, Patchouli, Gentle Healer, Freedom, Fortify

Joint Aches & Pains: Helichrysum, Spruce, Birch, Marjoram, Peppermint, Wintergreen, Relief, Sport Pro, Freedom Plus, True Blue, Soothing Relief, Migraine Relief

Joy: Bergamot, Orange, Cucumber, Awakening, Angel Assist, Rose, Love, Joyful, Mountain Retreat, Citrus Plus, Peaceful Moments

Kidneys: Fennel, Grapefruit, Juniper Berry, Rosemary, Sandalwood, Circle of Life, Vitality, Sport Pro, Freedom, True Blue, Fortify

Labor: Rose, Clary Sage, Frankincense, Jasmine, Lavender, Nutmeg, Baby Soft

Lack of Concentration: Focus, Brain Power, Grounding, Confidence

Lactation: Basil, Fennel, Anise, Jasmine, Dill

Laryngitis: Frankincense, Black Cumin, Rose, Sandalwood, Myrrh, Eucalyptus, Fortify, Freedom Plus, Confidence, Peaceful Moments

Laxative: Tangerine, Fennel, Anise, Black Cumin, Tummy Rub

Leg Cramps: Marjoram, Basil, Birch, Cypress, Ginger, Peppermint, Sports Pro, Relief, True Blue, Freedom Plus, Pain EZ, Soothing Relief

Leprosy: Frankincense, Black Cumin, Spice Traders

Lethargy: Rose, Jasmine, Potential, Love, Brain Power, Focus

Leukemia: Black Cumin, Frankincense

Leucorrhea (white vagina discharge): Black Cumin, Cedarwood, Eucalyptus, Frankincense, Hyssop, Lavender, Marjoram, Myrrh, Rosemary, Clary Sage, Sandalwood, Tea Tree

Libido: Rose, Neroli, Jasmine, Balance, Passion for Life, Citrus Plus, Love

Lice: Tea Tree, Eucalyptus, Black Cumin, Bug Free, Lavender, Lemongrass, Patchouli, Thyme,

Rosemary, Ravintsara, Neen Plus - Massage any of these oils into the hair and scalp, especially on the hairline of the neck, and leave on overnight. Wash all bedding in hot water.

Ligaments: Lemongrass, Citrus Plus (rebuild damaged tissue), Relief, Sport Pro, Freedom Plus, True Blue, Soothing Relief

Lipid Metabolism: Hyssop

Listlessness: Jasmine, Peppermint, Basil, Rosemary, Focus, Magnify, Balance, Love, Mountain Retreat

Liver: Carrot Seed, Black Cumin, Peppermint, Rosemary, Geranium, Grapefruit, Helichrysum, Juniper Berry, Myrtle, Circle of Life, Break Thru, Ravintsara, Tummy Rub, Rejuvenate

Loneliness: Rose, Mountain Retreat, Baby Soft, Love, Angel Assist, Gratitude, Calming, Citrus Plus, Peacemaker, Uplifting, Peaceful Moments

Loss of Appetite: Bay Leaf, Bergamot, Lime, Cardamom, Ginger, Myrrh, Black Pepper

Longevity: Fennel, Rosemary, Love, Fortify, Spice Traders, Exodus, Freedom Plus

Love: Lavender, Ylang Ylang, Rose Blend, Neroli Blend, Love, DNA Repair, Faith, Grateful, Uplifting, Passion for Life

Low Blood Pressure: Hyssop, Rosemary, Thyme, Circle of Life

Lumbago: Sandalwood, Thyme, Sport Pro, Relief, True Blue, Soothing Relief

Lungs: Ravintsara, Eucalyptus, Hyssop, Myrrh, Rosemary, Breathe EZ, Spice Traders, Freedom Plus, Resp EZ

Lupus: Black Cumin, Frankincense, Fortify,

Freedom Plus, Rejuvenate

Lymphatic System: Lavender, Lemon, Cypress, Frankincense, Grapefruit, Oregano, Gentle Healer, Freedom Plus, Vitality, Spice Traders, Rejuvenate, Citrus Plus

Lyme disease: Spruce, Peppermint, Black Cumin, Frankincense, Fortify, Freedom, Exodus, Spice Traders, Rejuvenate

MS: Clove Bud, Frankincense, Helichrysum, Black Cumin, Freedom Plus, Sport Pro, Relief, Soothing Relief, True Blue

Magnify Your Purpose: Myrrh, Rose Blend, Frankincense, Guardian, Magnify, Mountain Retreat, Faith, Angel Assist, Peacemaker

Malaria: Black Cumin, Eucalyptus, Oregano, Exodus, Spice Traders, Fortify, Freedom, Rejuvenate, Breathe EZ

Manic Depressant: Frankincense, Rose, Neroli, Balance, Break Thru, Confidence, Love, Calming, Serenity

Measles: Black Cumin, Lavender, Tea Tree, Eucalyptus, Freedom, Fortify, Spice Traders

Meditation: Cedarwood, Frankincense, Sandalwood, Rose, Dreamtime, Focus, Mountain Retreat, Balance, Love, Meditation

Memory: Basil, Cedarwood, Clove Bud, Lemon, Frankincense, Circle of Life, Focusing, Ginger, Rosemary, Peppermint

Menopause: Rose, Lavender, Chamomile, Clary Sage, Cypress, Fennel, Jasmine, Geranium, Sage, Hormone Balance, Freedom, Rejuvenate, Vitality

Menstruation: Chamomile (excessive), Cypress (excessive), Frankincense, Basil, Marjoram,

Rose (excessive), Peppermint, Lavender (pre), Hormone Balance, Rejuvenate, Freedom

Mental: Oregano (disease), Basil (fatigue), Eucalyptus (fatigue), Peppermint (fatigue), Petitgrain (clarity), Rosemary (fatigue), Ylang Ylang (fatigue), Focus, Brain Power

Metabolism: Oregano, Spearmint, Vitality

Mid-Life Crisis: Clary Sage, Hormone Balance, Confidence, Utopia, Balance, Support, Break Thru, In The Moment

Migraine: Basil, Eucalyptus, Lavender, Marjoram, Peppermint, Rosemary, Relief, Migraine Relief, True Blue, Soothing Relief, Brain Power, Freedom Plus

Mind: Rose, Basil, Rosemary, Lavender, Lemon, Peppermint, Frankincense, Focus, Confident, Brain Power, Fortify

Miscarriage: Utopia, Vitality, Rejuvenate, Confidence, Balance

Mononucleosis: Ravintsara, Fortify, Exodus, Spice Traders

Moodiness: Geranium, Lavender, Rosemary, Rose, Hormone Balance, Confidence, Love, Peacemaker, Citrus Plus, Peaceful Moments, Balance, Guardian

Motion Sickness: Ginger, Peppermint, Tummy Rub, Freedom Plus

Mosquito bites: Cedarwood, Lavender, Tea Tree, Purify, Freedom Plus, Bug Free

Mouth: Lavender (abscess), Bergamot (infections), Orange (ulcers), Tea Tree, Clove Bud, Freedom, Spice Traders, Fortify

Mucolytic: Hyssop, Rosemary, Orange

Mucus: See Catarrh

Muscles: Helichrysum, Marjoram, Rosemary, Freedom Plus, Relief, Sport Pro, Toning, True Blue, Soothing Relief, Nerve Repair

Muscular Dystrophy (MD): Marjoram, Birch, Peppermint, Sports Pro, Rejuvenate, Freedom Plus, True Blue, Soothing Relief

Myelin Sheath Damage: Helichrysum italicum, Gentle Healer, Freedom Plus, Nerve Repair

Nausea: Basil, Anise, Fennel, Ginger, Lavender, Peppermint, Spearmint, Tarragon, Tummy Rub, Freedom Plus

Nerves: Basil, Clove Bud (virus), Frankincense, Helichrysum italicum, Lavender, Marjoram, Melissa, Peppermint (stress), Rosemary, Gentle Healer, Grounding, Balance, Rejuvenate, Nerve Repair, Relief, Soothing Relief, True Blue

Nervous Exhaustion/Fatigue: Basil, Elemi, Eucalyptus, Ginger, Helichrysum italicum, Nerve Repair, Peppermint, Palmarosa, Rosemary, Relief, Rejuvenate, True Blue

Neuralgia/Sciatica: Marjoram, Helichrysum, Lavender, Peppermint, Sport Pro, Rosemary, Relief, Soothing Relief, True Blue

Neuromuscular: Helichrysum italicum, Clove Bud, Marjoram, Relief, Sport Pro, True Blue, Freedom Plus, Nerve Repair

Night Sweats: Sage, Hormone Balance

Nightmares: Lavender, Serenity, Calming, Dreamtime

Nose: Lemon (nosebleeds), Peppermint, Cypress, Rosemary, Lavender

Nursing/Lack of milk: Anise, Basil, Dill, Fennel

Obesity: Birch, Grapefruit, Fennel, Juniper Berry, Lemon, Orange, Mandarin, Tangerine, Cypress, Freedom Plus, Citrus Plus, Vitality, Rejuvenate, Toning, Slim and Trim

Odors: Cedarwood, Rosemary, Purify, Fortify

Oppressed Breathing: Basil, Rosemary, Peppermint, Eucalyptus, Focus, Breathe EZ, Resp EZ

Osteoporosis: Birch, Peppermint, Helichrysum, Relief, Freedom Plus, Sports Pro, True Blue

Ovaries: Myrtle, Rosemary, Hormone Balance, Vitality, Tummy Rub

Oxygen: Circle of Life, Brain Power, all the oils contribute to oxygenating the cells

Pain: Helichrysum, Birch, Clove, Spruce, Sport Pro, Pain EZ, Relief, Freedom Plus, True Blue, Nerve Repair, Soothing Relief, Migraine Relief

Palpitation: Orange, Ylang Ylang, Neroli, Rose Blend, Petitgrain, Circle of Life

Pancreas: Coriander, Helichrysum, Cypress, Dill, Vitality

Panic: Petitgrain, Confidence, Grounding

Para-Sympathetic System: Lemongrass, Marjoram, Freedom Plus, Nerve Repair

Parasites: Cinnamon Bark, Clove Bud, Hyssop, Oregano, Thyme, Tummy Rub, Freedom Plus

Parkinson's disease: Cedarwood, Myrrh, Sandalwood

Peace: Lavender, Orange, Rosewood, Rose, Angel Assist, Love, Mountain Breeze, Serenity, Peacemaker, DNA Repair, Uplifting, Calming, Peaceful Moments

Personal Growth: Rose, Angel Assist, Love, Magnify, Balance, Passion for Life, Confidence, Grateful, Uplifting,

Perspiration: Cedarwood, Lemongrass (excessive), Peppermint, Petitgrain (excessive)

Phlebitis: Helichrysum, Frankincense, Circle of Life, Confidence, Mountain Retreat, Serenity, Peaceful Moments, Soothing Relief

Physical: Cinnamon (energy), Lemon (energy), Coriander (exhaustion), Spice Traders, Fortify, Freedom, Rejuvenate, True Blue

Pineal Gland: Sandalwood, Frankincense, Cedarwood, Magnify, Brain Power, Balance, Serenity, Love, Confidence, Exodus

Pituitary Gland: Cedarwood, Sandalwood, Frankincense, (see Pineal Gland)

Plague: Black Cumin, Cinnamon Bark, Clove Bud, Oregano, Thyme, Exodus, Fortify, Spice Traders, Rejuvenate, Freedom Plus

Pleurisy: Black Cumin, Oregano, Peppermint, Marjoram, Rosemary, Eucalyptus, Marjoram, Hyssop, Exodus, Breathe EZ, Resp EZ, Fortify, Spice Traders, Rejuvenate, Freedom Plus

PMS: Clary Sage, Carrot Seed, Chamomile, Geranium, Lavender, Marjoram, Orange, Angel Assist, Hormone Balance, Rejuvenate

Pneumonia: Eucalyptus, Frankincense, Clove Bud, Hyssop, Cinnamon Bark, Oregano, Thyme, Exodus, Spice Traders, Breathe EZ. Fortify, Resp EZ, Rejuvenate

Poisoning: Cedarwood, Black Cumin, Juniper Berry, Tummy Rub, Rejuvenate, Freedom

Poison Ivy: Add Peppermint to rubbing alcohol - 10 to 50% Peppermint and 90 to 50% alcohol.

Another one I've heard is use chicken fat --- boil it down and then let it cool. Rub on area to take away itching.

Poor Circulation & Low Blood Pressure: Black Cumin, Cypress, Ginger, Lemon, Lemongrass, Black Pepper, Peppermint, Rosemary, Pine Needles, Oregano, Thyme, Circle of Life, First Aid, Freedom Plus, Cinnamon Blend, Soothing Relief, Rejuvenate

Pores: Lemongrass (open), Lavender, Chamomile, Rosewood, Ginger, Rose, Elemi, Skin Care, Baby Soft

Postnatal Depression: Rose, Frankincense, Sandalwood, Neroli, Confidence, Joyous, Love, Hormone Balance, Angel Assist, Peacemaker

Pregnancy: Geranium, Rose Blend, Baby Soft, Tummy Rub, Rejuvenate, Freedom Plus

Premature Aging: Myrrh, Frankincense, Rose, Elemi, Patchouli, Rosewood, Skin Care, Baby Soft, Freedom Plus, Toning, Sandalwood

Pride: Peppermint, Balance

Prosperity: Prosperity, Cinnamon Blend, Ginger, Patchouli, Bergamot

Prostate: Basil, Cypress, Black Cumin, Myrtle, Jasmine, Sandalwood, Spruce, Hormone Balance, Vitality

Protection: Black Cumin, Clove Bud, Guardian, Angel Assist, Mountain Retreat, Confidence, Love, Freedom Plus, Balance

Psoriasis: Bergamot, Cedarwood, Juniper Berry, Sandalwood, Carrot Seed, Chamomile, Lavender, Freedom Plus, Rejuvenate, Skin Care

Psychic Awareness: Rose, Jasmine, Cypress, Sandalwood, Eucalyptus, Lemongrass, Angel Assist, Balance, Blend, Mountain Retreat

Pulmonary: Cypress, Eucalyptus, Helichrysum, Hyssop, Sandalwood, Oregano (tuberculosis), Circle of Life, pH Balance

Purify: Purify, Eucalyptus, Fennel, Cinnamon Blend, Lemon, Lemongrass, Peppermint, Fortify, Gentle Healer, Joyous, Citrus Plus

Pyorrhea: Black Cumin, Cypress, Fortify, Frankincense, Freedom Plus

Radiation: Frankincense, Black Cumin, Fortify, Lavender, Gentle Healer (massage 10 days before & two weeks after radiation treatment), Oregano, Freedom Plus, Exodus, Rejuvenate

Rash: Tea Tree, Chamomile, Lavender, Black Cumin, Patchouli, Rosewood, Sandalwood, Baby Soft, Gentle Healer, Freedom Plus, Cucumber

Receding Gums: Tea Tree (brush teeth), Clove Bud, Spice Traders (brushing)

Regenerative: Black Cumin, Helichrysum, Geranium, Lavender, Lemongrass, Rosemary, Gentle Healer, Freedom Plus, Rejuvenate, Fortify, Exodus, Spice Traders, Toning

Relaxing: Lavender, Serenity, Citrus Plus, Mountain Retreat, Peaceful Moments, Calming

Resentment: Lemon, Rose, Forgiveness, Love, Break Thru, Confidence, Balance, Magnify

Respiratory System: Ravintsara, Black Cumin, Eucalyptus, Basil, Rosemary, Hyssop, Fortify, Spice Traders, Exodus, Breathe EZ, Resp EZ, Soothing Relief, Rejuvenate,

Restlessness: Lavender, Serenity, Confidence, Balance, Peaceful Moments, Citrus Plus

Restorative: Basil, Rosemary, Ravintsara, DNA

67

Repair, Rejuvenate, Uplifting, Nerve Repair

Rheumatism: Basil, Birch, Ginger, Marjoram, Helichrysum, Spruce, Black Pepper (rheumatoid arthritis), Freedom Plus, Relief, Soothing Relief, Sport Pro, True Blue, Migraine Relief

Rhinopharyngitis: Ravintsara, Fortify, Exodus, Spice Trader, Freedom Plus

Ringworm: Lavender, Myrrh, Black Cumin, Peppermint, Tea Tree, Gentle Healer, Freedom

Scabies: Bergamot, Lavender, Lemongrass, Peppermint, Spearmint, Pine Needles, Thyme, Rosemary, Freedom

Scalp Massage: Clary Sage, Holy Basil, Ylang Ylang, Sandalwood, Freedom, Hair Support

Scars: Helichrysum italicum & Florah Blend (best for healing scars), Frankincense, Rose, Rosewood, Lavender, Palmarosa, Patchouli, Sandalwood, Baby Soft, Skin Care

Sciatica: Spruce, Helichrysum, Lavender, Sandalwood, Relief, Sport Pro, Freedom Plus, Soothing Relief, (see Neuralgia)

Seasonal Affective Disorder: Balance, Confidence, Orange, Citrus Plus, Mountain Retreat, Peaceful Moments

Seborrhea: Patchouli, Rosemary, Freedom, Rejuvenate, Skin Care, Renew

Sedative: Chamomile, Lavender, Orange, Sandalwood, Serenity, Calming, Citrus Plus, Peaceful Moments

Self-Awareness: Orange, Balance, Love, Angel Assist, Magnify, Confidence, Uplifting

Self-Esteem: Geranium, Bergamot, Ylang Ylang, Rose, Sandalwood, Angel Assist, Love,

Confidence, Magnify, Balance, In The Moment, Guardian, DNA Repair, Grounding, Uplifting

Sensory System: Ginger, Peppermint

Sensitive Skin: Rose, Rosewood, Chamomile, Geranium, Skin Care, Balance (if one experiences a reaction to oils, use one drop on the crown and one drop on the navel)

Sesquiterpenes: Cedarwood, Myrtle, Ginger, Sandalwood, Frankincense, Black Pepper

Sexuality: Cinnamon Blend, Sandalwood, Patchouli, Geranium, In The Moments

Shingles: Ravintsara, Bergamot, Black Cumin, Eucalyptus, Breathe EZ, Freedom

Shock: Lavender, Melissa, Rosemary, Basil, Neroli, Peppermint, Focus, Brain Power

Sinus: Basil, Cedarwood, Clove, Eucalyptus, Myrtle, Respiratory EZ, Ravintsara, Rosemary, Breathe EZ, Break Thru, Freedom, Spice Traders, Sports Pro, Relief Me

Skeletal Disorders: Spruce, Rosewood, Frankincense, Birch, Confidence, Balance

Skin: Cucumber, Cedarwood (skin ulcers & skin diseases), Elemi, Frankincense, Patchouli, Rose, Ylang Ylang, Rosemary, Rosewood, Baby Soft (elasticity), Skin Care, Toning, Renew

Skunk Spray: One lady told me about using a 4 oz spray bottle of water with 10 drops of Lavender to spray over her dog several times after he had encountered a skunk. Purify may also work.

Sleep: Lavender, Chamomile, Serenity

Sluggishness: Eucalyptus, Peppermint, Lemon, Rosemary, Cypress, Focus, Rejuvenate

Smell: Basil, Peppermint, Focus, Rosemary

Smoking: Rejuvenate (stop), Support, Purify (odor), Bergamot (stop), Serenity, Circle of Life, Vitamin C is the best known substance to remove nicotine from the blood stream.

Snake bites: Basil, Cinnamon Bark, Clove Bud, Patchouli, Juniper Berry, Oregano, Freedom, Purify, Spice Traders

Solar Plexus: Spruce, Magnify, Rosemary (energizes), Freedom Plus

Sore Throat: Black Cumin, Ginger, Eucalyptus, Hyssop, Oregano, Tea Tree, Fortify, Exodus, Spice Traders, Freedom Plus

Spasms: Birch, Peppermint, Spruce, Marjoram, Lavender, Freedom Plus, Relief, Soothing Relief, Sport Pro, True Blue, Migraine Relief

Speaking: Geranium (fear), Rose, Angel Assist, Confidence, Magnify, Mountain Retreat

Spiritual Awareness: Frankincense, Myrrh, Rose, Angel Assist, Confidence, Mountain Retreat, Balance, In The Moment, Love

Spleen: Fennel, Helichrysum, Fortify, Exodus, Freedom Plus, Spice Traders

Spots: Bergamot, Helichrysum, Cypress, Tea Tree, Eucalyptus, Lavender, Citrus Plus, Circle of Life, Cucumber, Renew

Sprains: Birch, Clove, Eucalyptus, Helichrysum, Basil, Marjoram, Rosemary, Pain EZ, Relief, Sport Pro, Freedom Plus, True Blue

Stabilizing: Frankincense, Spruce, Rosemary, Peppermint, Lavender, Confidence, Balance, In The Moments, Mountain Retreat

Staphylococci: Black Cumin, Cinnamon Blend, Clove Bud, Oregano, Thyme, Spice Traders, Exodus, Fortify,

Sterility: Geranium, Balance

Stiffness: Marjoram, Birch, Peppermint, Spruce, Sport Pro, Freedom Plus, Relief, Revitalize, True Blue, Pain EZ, Soothing Relief

Stimulant: Lime, Peppermint, Rosemary, Focus, Rejuvenate, Freedom, First Aid

Stings: Purify, Freedom Plus, Basil, Black Cumin, Juniper Berry, Lavender, Relief, Gentle Healer, Pain EZ, Helichrysum

Stomach: Helichrysum, Black Cumin, Ginger, Peppermint, Tummy Rub, Freedom Plus

Strains: Peppermint, Basil, Birch, Lemongrass, Marjoram, Sport Pro, Relief, Nerve Repair

Strengthening: Confidence, Rejuvenate, Freedom Plus, Mountain Retreat, Grounding

Stress: Cedarwood, Frankincense, Geranium, Helichrysum, Rosemary, Rosewood, Serenity, Confidence, Citrus Plus, Balance, Love

Stretch Marks: Lavender, Myrrh, Baby Soft (apply during pregnancy), Freedom Plus, Toning

Stuttering: Serenity

Subconscious: Helichrysum, Focus, Balance, Angel Assist, DNA Repair, Brain Power

Sunburn: Chamomile, Lavender, Tea Tree, Freedom, Relieve the Heat

Supportive: Myrrh, Frankincense, Black Cumin, Spruce, Confidence, Angel Assist, Balance, Angel Assist, Magnify, Guardian, Love

Suicidal: Rose, Sandalwood, Frankincense,

Love, Balance, Uplifting, Utopia, Grateful

Swelling: Peppermint, Basil, Birch, Sports Pro, Wintergreen, Relief, Freedom Plus, Pain EZ, Nerve Repair, Helichrysum

Tachycardia: Lavender, Ylang Ylang, Freedom Plus

Teething Pains: Chamomile, Clove Bud, Spice Traders, Freedom Plus, Fortify – these all need to be diluted for a baby

Temper: Rose, Balance, Confidence, Break Thru, Serenity, Citrus Plus

Temperature (body): Peppermint - one drop in 16 ounces of water

Tendons & Joints: Lemongrass, Peppermint, Chamomile, Basil, Birch, Freedom Plus, Relief, Sport Pro, Toning, Soothing Relief, True Blue

Tension: Basil, Lavender, Chamomile, Ylang Ylang, Frankincense, Spice Traders, Confidence

Testicles: Rosemary

Testosterone: Sage

Throat: Black Cumin, Ginger, Hyssop, Tea Tree, Myrrh, Lemon (infection), Peppermint (infection), Freedom Plus, Fortify, Spice Traders

Thrush: Bergamot, Black Cumin, Geranium, Myrrh, Lavender, Tea Tree, Freedom, Fortify

Thymus: Spruce, Black Cumin, Balance, Rejuvenate, Freedom Plus, Fortify

Thyroid Dysfunction: Clove Bud, Myrtle, Freedom Plus, Vitality

Ticks: Lemongrass, Marjoram, Peppermint, Tea Tree, Purify, Freedom Plus

Tinnitus: Basil, Helichrysum, Black Cumin, Peppermint, Fortify, Rejuvenate, Nerve Repair – **never put directly in ear** - put on finger tip or cotton ball and apply to ear

Tissue: Cypress (tightens), Geranium (tightens), Helichrysum (repair), Patchouli (repair), Relief, Tea Tree (repair), Lemongrass (toner), Petitgrain (regeneration), Freedom Plus, Gentle Healer, (regeneration), Citrus Plus, Rejuvenate

Tonic: Oregano, Rejuvenate

Tonsillitis: Black Cumin, Hyssop, Peppermint, Lavender, Rosemary, Myrtle, Tea Tree, Thyme, Spice Traders, Fortify, Freedom Plus

Toothache: Clove Bud, Peppermint, Tea Tree, Spice Traders (use for brushing teeth), Relief, Sport Pro, Myrrh, Freedom Plus

Tooth Decay: Clove Bud, Spice Traders

Touchiness: Lemon, Rose, Geranium, Love, Magnify, Break Thru, Balance, Confidence

Toxins: See Detoxifies

Transition: Cypress, Love, Angel Assist, In The Moment, Balance, Confidence, Uplifting

Tranquilizing: Valerian, Serenity, Utopia, Citrus Plus, Peaceful Moments, Peacemaker

Tremors: Marjoram, Basil, Freedom Plus

Tropical Infection: Black Cumin, Cinnamon Bark, Tea Tree, Gentle Healer, Freedom Plus, Exodus, Spice Traders, Fortify

Tuberculosis: Clove Bud, Tea Tree, Hyssop, Frankincense, Rejuvenate, Oregano, Thyme, Breathe EZ, Fortify, Exodus, Spice Traders

Tumor: Black Cumin, Clove Bud, Frankincense, Lemon, Freedom Plus

Twitching muscles: Basil, Marjoram, Nerve Repair, Freedom Plus, Relief, True Blue, Sports Pro, Freedom Plus, Soothing Relief, True Blue

Typhoid: Cinnamon Bark, Oregano, Black Cumin, Fortify, Rejuvenate, Exodus

Ulcers: Black Cumin, Cedarwood (skin ulcers), Eucalyptus, Geranium, Juniper Berry, Lavender, Tummy Rub

Uplifting: Frankincense, Elemi, Rose, Neroli, Orange, Joyous, Mountain Retreat, Peaceful Moments, Balance, Grateful, Citrus Plus

Urinary System: Black Cumin, Cedarwood, Frankincense, Thyme, Exodus, Freedom Plus, Spice Traders, Rejuvenate, Fortify

Uterus: Jasmine, Frankincense, Thyme, Myrtle, Hormone Balance, Baby Soft

Vaginal Thrush: Tea Tree, Myrrh, Bergamot, Spice Traders, Exodus, Fortify

Vaginitis: Rosemary, Frankincense, Geranium, Lavender, Petitgrain, Confidence

Varicose Veins: Cypress, Helichrysum, Circle of Life, Freedom Plus – by adding a few drops each of Circle of Life, Rejuvenate, Cypress, and Freedom Plus you may have better results..

Vascular System: Bergamot (ulcers), Cypress (veins), Lemon (veins), Lemongrass (veins & walls), Peppermint (veins), Rosemary (veins), Circle of Life, Freedom

Vertigo: Lavender, Peppermint, Melissa, Neroli

Viral Colitis: Helichrysum, Black Cumin, Exodus, Rosewood, Oregano, Fortify

Viruses: Cinnamon Bark, Clove Bud, Black Cumin, Melissa, Oregano, Palmarosa, Exodus, Rosemary, Fortify, Ravintsara, Spice Traders

Visualization: Elemi, Angel Assist, Magnify, Love, Balance, Serenity, Dreamtime, Meditation, Grateful, Mountain Retreat, Uplifting

Vitality: Vetiver, Vitality

Vomiting: Black Cumin, Fennel, Peppermint, Freedom Plus, Tummy Rub (see Nausea)

Warts: Cinnamon Bark, Tea Tree, Black Cumin, Oregano, Thyme, Lemon, Lime, or Fortify on wart and Love over the heart

Wasp Stings: Juniper Berry, Tea Tree, Purify, Lavender, Purify, Relief, Gentle Healer

Water Retention: Tangerine, Orange, Juniper Berry, Cypress, see Edema

Weak Cell Walls: Fortify, Freedom Plus, Circle of Life, Rejuvenate, Toning

Weight Loss: Grapefruit, Patchouli, Thyme, Vitality, Love, Toning, Slim and Trim

Whooping Cough: Basil, Cypress, Tea Tree, Black Cumin, Helichrysum, Marjoram, Oregano, Rosemary, Thyme, Fortify, Breathe EZ, Exodus, Freedom Plus, Spice Traders

Willpower: Marjoram, Rose, Magnify, Confidence, Uplifting, Grounding, Meditation

Womb: Myrrh, Baby Soft, Love, Citrus Plus

Worms: Black Cumin, Oregano, Cinnamon Bark, Tummy Rub, Freedom

Wounds: Helichrysum, Lavender, Tea Tree, Clove Bud, Frankincense, Cypress, Gentle Healer, Relief, Freedom Plus, Soothing Relief

Wrinkles: Myrrh, Patchouli, Rose, Sandalwood, Frankincense, Elemi, Cucumber, Skin Care,

Freedom, Baby Soft, Toning, Renew

~~~~~~~~~~

When you have used an oil and are not receiving the benefits you wish, switch to another one. Everyone is so different. Your body chemistry may work better with a different oil. Another thing to consider is the pain may be an emotion seeking to be released. The benefits of essential oils for emotions are almost immediate. Just sitting and breathing in the oils bring benefits of relieving stress, anger, frustration, and emotional blocks. They bring feelings of peace, joy and serenity.

As you start using the essential oils, experiment with them for various uses and you will soon find many more applications. Add your findings to your notebook and, whenever possible, share your new knowledge with others. Remember, the use of essential oils is relatively new even though they have been around for thousands of years. Since there has been very little research on the essential oils, many of their healing properties are still unknown. At present time, research companies find it unprofitable to do the research because the oils cannot be patented.

If you have had some experiences with the essential oils that you would like to share I would love hearing about them. With your permission I would like to share your experience with others in my classes or in the newsletter. This is the way we can all learn from each other. My email address is Bevonne25@yahoo.com. Please mention in the subject line your email is about liquid copals or essential oils so I don't inadvertently delete it.

SUGGESTED WAYS TO USE THE ESSENTIAL OILS

When you share your knowledge of the essential oils it seems your mind is open to new ways of using them. But then you hoard your knowledge you seem to lose it. Over the years I have learned from many people and you will too. Those who generously share their knowledge and talents to reach out and touch others' lives for good are what make life so beautiful. This section contains various ways I have learned to use and apply the oils.

Remember, these are only suggestions. Since copals work with all healing modalities, you will learn how to adapt these suggestions to fit your own healing style. Sometimes you will be unable to do a full technique on a person. Remember, just putting one essential oil on or having them smell an oil, is better than not sharing with them at all.

One way of applying the oils to be beneficial is the Vita Flex Technique. Vita Flex means vitality through the reflexes. Here is a modified version to use on the bottom of the feet when applying the essential oils. To learn more read Stanley Burroughs book, Healing for the Age of Enlightenment. To see the Vita Flex Technique go to my Rejuvenation Training DVD. When combining the healing frequency of the oils and that of the person applying them, this application creates rapid and phenomenal results. Remember, the activating force of all healing is the energy of love.

BASIC VITA FLEX APPLICATION
When applied through specific hand rotation movements, a vibrational healing energy is released as the fingernails come in contact with the reflex points. The energy flows into the neuro electrical pathways through the body. The sole of the foot contains 200,000 sensory nerve endings, more than any other part of the body. The following are the steps I use:

Step I: Spread a small hand towel under the feet to protect the floor.

Step 2: Rub 3 to 6 drops (depending on the size of the foot) of Confidence on bottom of each foot.

Step 3: Starting on the heel of the right foot, place the tips of your fingers of the left hand on the bottom of the right foot near the **outer** edge. Press lightly and roll onto the fingernails. Keeping your fingers in contact with the right foot, move your left hand down the foot towards the toes about a finger width and press lightly and roll onto the fingernails again. Repeat this process all the way to the toes 3 times making sure you go over the same area. Now move towards the center of the foot one-finger width and repeat the process in this area 3 times before moving again a finger width in and repeating 3 times. (I will usually switch hands and finish the right foot using my right hand. It's easier for me to do the whole foot this way.)

Continue this process until you have covered the entire right foot. Then move to the **inside** of the left foot. Start again with your left hand at the heel as you work down the foot toward the big toe with the same rolling action. Work across the foot from right to left using the rolling action 3 times in each area. Keep as straight in front of the feet as possible for better energy flow.

Step 4: Hold feet (right hand to right foot and left hand to left foot) for 3 to 10 minutes or until you feel an energy exchange. This feels like a strong heart beat in your hands. You are assisting to balance the body.

Step 5: You may wish to apply another oil and repeat the process.

You can find a variety of foot, ear and spine charts on the internet. Find the ones you would like to learn from. By studying the charts it will help find various ways and areas to apply the essential oils. The charts are just another tool to help you see how unique the body is. You will learn that by massaging certain areas on the feet, ear, or back it will help other areas to heal.

Here is some interesting information about massaging the ears. The ears, like the hands and feet, have reflexes that affect the entire body. These important reflexes may stimulate a renewed flow of life-force energy into every part of your body when pressed, pulled and massaged. The ear chart shows very accurately the mental and physical condition of the individual.

Because of the relationship of the reflexes in the ears to the rest of the body, reflex massage of the ears can be of assistance in correcting many symptoms of malfunctioning organs. The ear is a complex sense organ endowed with many pressure points. This allows us to use the fingers to stimulate these sensitive reflexes. People twist, pull and pinch their ears unconsciously, especially the earlobes, when something perplexing bothers them. Thus, instinctively, people are using this wonderful healing technique.

If a certain point in the ear is painful to the touch, it may mean there is a health concern in some other area of the body. The pain may actually be calling for assistance. Somewhere the body is not getting its full supply of energy. By pressing the tender reflex in the ear, especially if you have applied essential oils such as lavender to the ear first, you are contacting another main circuit that will assist to open up the line to full power. Because there are some 100 reflexes in the ears, it is almost impossible to pinpoint them all.

My favorite way is to apply the oil over the entire ear. Such a small and simple application benefits the whole body. Place the fingers behind the ears and flatten them forward against the side of the head. Hold the ear with the third, fourth and fifth fingers. Tap the index finger on the ear to get a drum sound. Doing this about five times may assist to stimulate the gall bladder.

Now, place the cupped hand over one ear and tap gently with the other hand to get the sound of a seashell. This may stimulate the kidneys and the triple-warmer organs.

While doing both ears at the same time, start at the top and pinch the ear between the thumb and forefinger. Do this part of the ears several times. Your client should notice the ears beginning to tingle and warm. Using this same technique of massage, pull, tug, and pinch the lower lobes for a few seconds. After this, start at the top of the ear and pinch and roll the outer ridge all the way around to the lobes. Now hook the little fingers in the holes of the ears and pull out in all directions. End this massage by pinching and massaging the small flap located in front of the ear opening.

Now press the reflex points just behind the lobes of the ears. Press first on the bony section and then in the hollow. These are magic reflex points that may free you from tension, headaches, and improve sinuses. One simple method that may assist to bring back hearing is to apply Helichrysum italicum to the end of the fourth fingers (the ring fingers). Press the ends of the fingers together for several minutes at a time, several times a day. This has been known to relieve an earache.

By working on the entire outer ear (rubbing and pinching), circulation is increased over the entire body. Use Lavender or an oil of your choice that has been diluted. There are many reflex points on the outer ear and at the entrance to the ear canal that produce good results all over the body.

This is a quick way to warm up on a cold day.

THE CRANE EXERCISE

This is a good example of how to use the essential oils in applications you come across in your reading. I discovered an interesting book hidden away on a basement shelf called <u>The Crane Exercise</u> by Stephen T. Chang, M.D. It explains a simple method to not only lose weight and inches but to promote proper digestion, sound sleep, and a healthy heart. Using several liquid copals with this technique has been beneficial in enhancing the process. This method comes from the ancient Chinese healers.

The Crane Exercise was named after the crane that appears to be constantly stimulating its abdominal area as it stands and alternately folds first one leg and then the other into its belly. The exercise is designed to make the internal organs more effective.

As we get older, exercising the stomach and abdominal area becomes more difficult. The abdominal area seems to be the one-place deposits of various fatty tissues like to accumulate. The excessive weight brings on mental and physical fatigue. The shift of weight to the lower front of the body puts stress on the spine, often causing lower back pain. This effortless two-minute exercise consists of two parts. It is simple yet effective.

First, begin by lying flat on your back and relaxing. Apply two or three drops of oil on your abdomen and massage in a circular motion. Next rub your hands together until warm. Put the palm of your predominate hand (if you are right handed, use your right hand) on your navel.

Start to rub clockwise from the center, first in small circles, and then gradually expand the movement until the upper and lower limits of the stomach and abdomen are being massaged. When you have completed the first movement,

reverse it, rubbing counterclockwise in smaller and smaller circles until you are back to the center of the navel.

Rub slowly and with gentle pressure. Repeat this motion as long as you feel comfortable, or have time to do so, but for at least two minutes.

Part two is using your body energy and visualization techniques. Your body is electrical. The gentle rubbing in ever-widening circles actually causes energy to flow from your hand through the skin to gently brush with energy the cells and tissues throughout the stomach area. Visualizing this energy process actually increases the effectiveness of the exercise.

In the first part of the exercise, the electricity from your own hand gently massages the intestines, the blood vessels, and the digestive and eliminatory systems. Fatty accumulations and deposits are disturbed from their resting-places and eventually broken up. They are then passed into the eliminatory system and out of the body. Your stomach and abdomen are literally rubbed away!

When you rub in a clockwise direction, you are encouraging proper bowel movements. Quite often constipation and being over weight are symptoms indicating that the digestive and eliminatory organs have become lazy, obstructed, or de-energized. Using the copals with this exercise would be very beneficial. Tummy Rub, Ginger, Peppermint, Fennel, Nutmeg, Slim & Trim, or Freedom Plus would be good choices to rub over the stomach and abdomen area before starting this exercise.

The clockwise motion also stimulates the peristaltic activity of the intestine and slows the water removal process down to normal levels so the food doesn't become compacted and cause constipation. Rubbing in a counterclockwise motion has the opposite effect and is beneficial for chronic diarrhea. It helps to solidify fecal material as it passes through the intestine. This rubbing action has been known to assist chronic diarrhea.

If chronic constipation or diarrhea is not your problem, but being overweight is, then it is necessary to incorporate both movements along with visualization into the rubbing sequence. Remember, losing weight is largely a matter of increasing the efficiency of the digestive organs. If food is not processed in the body properly, it hardly matters what or how much you eat. Have you ever tried eating less or changing your diet and still found yourself unable to lose weight? This may be because your digestive and elimination processes are not what they should be.

When food assimilation and elimination is ineffective or obstructed, a significant portion of what you eat tends to be stored for very long periods of time in the body. The Crane Exercise is like a natural colonic irrigation. If you are willing to do the exercise regularly two times a day for two weeks, you will begin to see results.

The first part of the exercise is rubbing. The second, and equally important part, is concentrating on the feeling of warmth within the area being massaged. When you feel warmth, no matter how small it may be, excess fat is being burned off around the stomach and intestines, metabolized, then discarded.

The two important points are to rub lightly and concentrate on feeling warmth and energy as your hand moves over the entire area. The key is the energy not the pressure. If you have trouble concentrating, you may want to use the oils of Focus, Magnify, or Confidence first across your forehead, on your ears and the back of your neck before you begin the exercise.

There are various ways for you to visualize this

technique. You can imagine energy coming from your hand, brushing the skin and organs before going deeper and deeper into the body. Another way is to imagine a small fire in the stomach that grows larger and larger as you rub. Or imagine a small dot of blue, green, yellow or white (the healing colors) in the center of your abdomen that grows larger and goes deeper into the skin as you gently rub. You will soon feel actual warmth where at first you only imagined it.

Doing this exercise regularly twice a day will bring other benefits as well. Your digestion will improve and you may notice an upswing in your level of vitality. Halitosis can be eliminated and the blood vessels will be gradually strengthened. When you rub your abdominal area, blood is drawn away from the head and brain usually shutting down the mental chatter allowing you to drift into a restful sleep.

DIFFUSING ESSENTIAL OILS
Diffusing essential oils is a very beneficial way to use them. Not only is the fragrance uplifting and pleasant, but this method allows the oils to enter quickly into the body through the nose. All essential oils have very positive aromatic influences on the body.

There are three things to look for in a diffuser: 1) no metal parts, 2) the copals stay away from anything electrical and 3) no heat is used. Using metal or heat can alter the healing energies or the chemical makeup of the oils.

The diffuser I use actually screws the bottle of essential oil into the non-metal diffusing top and sits in a base. When I want to change the copal being diffused, I simply unscrew the diffusing top and place it on another oil bottle. It is very quick, simple and there's no wasting the essential oils trying to get them out of the diffuser and back into the bottle.

When traveling and unable to use a diffuser, fill a

4-ounce spray bottle with water and add 15 to 20 drops of the essential oil. Just remember to shake the bottle a few times before spraying. When I travel I like to take one bottle of Purify to use in hotel rooms to purify the air and bed.

SWEATING TO ENHANCE A CLEANSE

When I talk about sweating it doesn't mean the kind you do from exercise. The type of sweating for cleansing is done in your own bath tub with hot water. Your skin is the largest elimination organ of your body and plays a very important part in removing toxins. By taking "hot" baths with various oils - ginger, salt, baking soda or vinegar the body eliminates toxic build-up. Sweating is an important part of cleansing. When hot sweating baths are taken 5 to 6 times a week, the elimination of toxins through the skin takes the burden off the liver and GI tract.

Cleansing the body on the inside is a way to rebuild or improve your health. Before you start a cleanse it is important that the channels the body uses to clear the toxins be functioning properly. The major channels the body uses for cleansing are the skin, liver, intestinal tract and lungs. When these are blocked and you start a cleanse, it will only add more stress to your body, causing fatigue, headaches, sore throat, or other flu-like symptoms. If you are doing a major detoxifying program it is beneficial to continue the 5 to 6 hot baths a week for at least 8 weeks and then reduce to 4 a week for several more weeks.

The water for a "sweating bath" needs to feel hot rather than warm. As you start filling the bath add the salt, Ginger, or essential oils and then climb in. You will be able to get the water hotter as you gradually get use to it. It takes the body about 10 minutes to start sweating. You will feel your forehead getting hot and sweaty. You should continue sweating for 15 to 20 minutes minimum. The baths usually last 25 to 30 minutes or longer. Relax and take some time for yourself. It has probably been years since you have spent time relaxing in the tub.

For years I have used "Hot Ginger Baths" for my children when they would get sick. I found that if I used two tablespoons of powdered Ginger in a tub of hot water at the very beginning of an illness, it was usually gone by the next morning. I like doing the hot bath at night so I can wrap in a sheet, get under the covers, and continue sweating. It is best to wrap in an old sheet because some of the toxins being released will stain.

Remember, sweating is the key. Sweating from exercise is not the same as the sweating that occurs during a hot bath. In a hot bath the heat comes from outside the body going to the core of the body releasing toxins stored deeper within. Only sweating induced by a hot bath will work effectively to deeply detoxify the body.

Some of the essential oils used to detoxify are Ginger, Juniper Berry, Grapefruit, Black Cumin, Fennel, Rosemary, Fortify, Patchouli, Basil, and Lemon. When you are using "hot" oils use only 6 drops in you bath. Here are some bath suggestions from Europe.

BATH-BALNEO THERAPY

Essential Oils are used in many European Spas.
Add the oils to a large glass of milk before
pouring in bath.

Muscle Pain Bath
7 drops Juniper Berry
5 drops Lavender
6 drops Rosemary

Stimulating Bath
4 drops Rosemary
4 drops Orange
4 drops Jasmine

Refreshing Bath
5 drops Bergamot
2 drops Geranium
2 drops Lavender
5 drops Lemongrass

Anti-Inflammation
8 drops Lavender
3 drops Lemon
8 drops Tea Tree

Head Ache Relief
10 drops Lavender
2 drops Peppermint
4 drops Lemon

Anti-Stress Bath
6 drops Lavender
2 drops Marjoram
2 drops Ylang Ylang

Cleansing Bath
2 drops Lavender
2 drops Thyme
2 drops Sage
2 drops Eucalyptus
2 drops Cypress
2 drops Myrtle
2 drops Geranium

Relaxing Bath
8 drops Geranium
6 drops Lemon
4 drops Clary Sage

Children's Bath
5 drops Lavender
5 drops Orange
1 drop Chamomile

Common Cold Bath
5 drops Lavender
3 drops Myrtle
5 drops Pine
1 drop Peppermint
1 drop Thyme

Anti-Depressant Bath
1 drop Thyme
7 drops Lavender
3 drops Rosemary
2 drops Sage
2 drops Juniper Berry

Relaxing Bath
5 drops Clary Sage
2 drops Lavender
2 drops Ylang Ylang
1 drop Vetiver

Anti-Rheumatic Bath
1 drop Thyme
5 drops Rosemary
5 drops Eucalyptus or Tea Tree
5 drops Lavender

Sensual Bath
4 drops Cypress
2 drops Geranium
6 drops Sandalwood

SYSTEMS of the BODY

I have enjoyed doing this section and learning how the body works. When we build health we need to work on all levels of our being. I am always amazed at how much abuse our bodies can take and still keep serving us to the best of their ability. We are wonderful!

As you look at yourself, determine which of your systems needs improvement and is being affected by your life style. Then use the essential oils that may help benefit those systems. Although the systems are presented separately, it is important to keep in mind that all the systems, structures and functions, are closely coordinated and integrated. The lists are to assist you in choosing which oil may be most beneficial. In selecting which oil to use, refer to the Single and Synergies Essential Oil sections for more information and go with your feelings. Again, the essential oils are not listed in any certain order; they are just some of the ones known to benefit that system.

In my research, it was interesting to learn that all the minerals are needed for each system of the body. Remember the Minerals, Enzymes, Probiotics, Ageless Plus, and Nature's Nutrients will benefit the whole body.

CIRCULATORY

Circle of Life	Focus	Fir
Geranium	Nutmeg	Ginger
Chamomile	Clove Bud	Lemon
Mt. Savory	Cypress	Basil
Eucalyptus	Ylang Ylang	Thyme
Freedom Plus	Lavender	Hyssop
Helichrysum	Cedarwood	Birch
Juniper Berry	Orange	Marjoram
Lemongrass	Peppermint	Rosemary
Black Pepper	Sandalwood	Rose
Tangerine	Sport Pro	

The heart is a highly effective muscular pump, the powerhouse behind the circulatory system, and the means by which blood is transported around the body. Rose Blend, Circle of Life, Ylang Ylang, Orange and minerals are good choices. The blood carries nutrients and oxygen to all the tissues of the body and then carries waste products away from the tissues.

Arteries, which carry blood away from the heart, are the highway along which all the nutrients necessary for growth, repair and maintenance of the body's cells are carried. The arteries divide and sub-divide, eventually flowing into millions of microscopic capillaries which permeate all our tissues. This is where the nutrients are delivered and waste products are received. The blood then returns through the veins to the heart.

The transport of oxygen and carbon dioxide between the lungs and tissues is dependent not only on the condition of the heart, arteries and veins, but also on the health of the blood itself. Lemon oil has been known to assist in stimulating red and white blood cell formation.

Using oils such as Circle of Life, Cypress, Black Pepper, Nutmeg or Ginger in a massage, on the ears or in a warm bath, may stimulate poor circulation. When essential oils are in the bath water they are also carried into the body. Deep breathing assists the healthy return of the blood to the heart through the veins.

For varicose veins, practice deep, abdominal breathing and a gentle massage of the affected area with the oils of Cypress and Circle of Life. Always massage upward, towards the heart when working on varicose veins.

The two major factors causing high blood pressure may be stress and arteriosclerosis.

79

Both are avoidable. Relaxation and diet may play a major part in reducing blood pressure. In high blood pressure, the body needs to rid itself of excess fluids. Tangerine, Cedarwood or Patchouli may assist you in this. These oils reduce both stress and excess fluids. Essential oils and the minerals that are beneficial for high blood pressure are Lemon, Hyssop, Ylang Ylang and potassium.

DIGESTIVE

Anise Seed	Black Cumin	Basil
Cardamom	Bay Leaf	Ginger
Clove Bud	Peppermint	Lemon
Coriander	Tummy Rub	Fennel
Frankincense	Thyme	Geranium
Lavender	Tarragon	Grapefruit
Juniper Berry	Tangerine	Myrrh
Lemongrass	Marjoram	Nutmeg
Orange	Oregano	Patchouli
Black Pepper	Rosemary	Spearmint
Melaleuca	Freedom Plus	Stevia
Enzymes	Probiotics	

Through the middle of the body runs a hollow tube which is the digestive tract. It is lined with mucus membrane. Different parts secrete the digestive juices required to break down the food into assumable form. Digestion is the chemical process by which the proteins, fats and carbohydrates of food are broken down into smaller, chemical units that are capable of being absorbed into the body.

The process of digestion starts when food is chewed and mixed with saliva. Inflammation of the gums is quite common and has been completely healed by using a drop or two of Tea Tree or Spice Traders on the toothbrush along with the regular toothpaste when brushing your teeth. People have also reported using the Tea Tree has helped whiten their teeth.

The muscular tube conveys chewed food to the stomach where it is added to and mixed with acid and digestive enzymes. The stomach converts food into a form the body can use. The partially digested food moves to the small intestine where bile and more enzymes are added. The enzymes come from the pancreas and the bile from the gall bladder. Bile is made by the liver and stored (between meals) in the gall bladder. The bile contains chemicals that are needed for the absorption of fats. Digestion and absorption is a slow and complex process. Over 20 feet of small intestine permits these vital functions to be carried out before the residue of waste material enters the large intestine.

The fluid mixed with the digested food is reabsorbed in the large intestine. When the re-absorption of fluid is complete, the final residue of fecal material passes into the rectum for excretion. Elimination is a vital function of the digestive tract, for in addition to voiding the residue of food and fluids, the intestines must also rid the body of other waste products. If the excretion is impaired, a build-up of toxic waste will result. The health of the colon and its regular peristaltic movements and evacuation are dependent on a diet containing plenty of fiber which stimulates contractions.

Proper digestive functioning also depends on nervous control. When a meal is eaten, the autonomic nervous system sends more bile to the digestive system. The nervous system also governs the secretion of hydrochloric acid in the stomach. When treating digestive problems, it is good to use Chamomile or Ginger to relax the nervous system as well as acting directly on the digestion.

The liver is the largest organ and main chemical workshop of the body. It plays a vital role in maintaining health and overcoming disease. Besides making bile, the liver performs hundreds of other complex processes required for life. All the food products absorbed through the wall of the small intestine are carried directly to the liver by a separate blood system, the portal vein. In the liver, these chemical substances are either used to make other chemical materials needed by the body (as blood proteins) or are stored in such a way as to be available for later use.

Because of the liver's central role in cleansing the body, it is important when treating chronic disease to regulate its functions. In the spring it is good to clear out the residue of heavy winter meals. For those who have been taking chemical drugs over a period of time, a liver-cleansing program may be essential. In the make-up of some oils, such as Birch and Wintergreen, are toxic chemicals. These toxic chemicals may store in the liver and build up over time. For those who use these and other copals on a regular basis, it would be beneficial to do a liver cleanse yearly.

There are several things you can do to help heal the liver. The first is to stop overworking it by changing the way you eat. Rest your digestive tract by eating small meals so the body will not have to use a lot of energy for digestion. Drink plenty of lemon water and sip vegetable soups or fresh vegetable juices. Eliminate animal foods completely while you are cleansing because the weakened liver cannot handle ammonia, a by-product of protein digestion. Stay away from cooking oils and butter because they slow down the liver function. Eat lightly steamed foods. Eat chlorophyll-rich greens and as much raw food as you can. Your last meal of the day should be a light one, taken early enough that the stomach is completely empty before you go to sleep.

Other ways you can help the liver is to exercise daily and get more rest; however, avoid lying down right after eating a meal if you have over eaten. You need to expend energy until you burn off that excess food. Hospital records show that most gall bladder patients are overweight. The diet should be mostly raw and cooked vegetables, vegetable juices and moderate amounts of fruits and seeds.

Diarrhea is usually caused by an infection or irritation of the digestive tract and is often accompanied by nausea and vomiting which is the normal way the body eliminates poisons. Once you have determined there is no serious cause, you should allow the condition to run its course, being sure to replace lost fluids and electrolytes. I learned the following formula when we lived in Africa. In one-quart of water mix 8 teaspoons sugar, ½ teaspoon salt and 8 drops of the lemon essential oil. Do not leave the sugar out because it is important for absorption. Drink one 8 ounce glass every few hours.

Infants may quickly collapse after bouts of diarrhea and vomiting if lost fluids and electrolytes are not promptly replaced. The minerals of calcium, potassium, germanium or a complete mineral supplement will assist in restoring the electrolytes. When experiencing diarrhea you should avoid cold drinks and cold food since digestive activity is aided by warmth. Nausea has been known to respond well to the spice copals of Ginger, Peppermint, Cinnamon Bark and Clove Buds.

Constipation is usually the result of poor diet and lack of exercise. Use a cleansing program and drink plenty of water (a minimum of half your body weight in ounces a day). Using Tummy Rub on the bottom of the feet and over the whole abdominal area may assist with constipation. I suggest diluting the Tummy Rub with carrier oil when doing the stomach area since some of the oils in this blend are considered hot. The MSM and the Crain Exercise mentioned in this book have also been known to help constipation. Good health is a result of proper digestion. If you aren't digesting your food properly, you have fermentation. If you have body odor, you are not eliminating or digesting properly. Enzymes may be of benefit here since it is believed the cause of degenerative diseases is the lack of enzymes. Toxic chemicals are stored in the fat of the body. Enzymes from the raw food we eat break down toxins and build the digestive system.

To be healthy you need a healthy colon. Raw fruits, vegetables, grains, nuts and seeds will provide bulk and enzymes for better health. I like the saying "dead foods – dead body, live foods – live body." A food is considered "dead" when it is cooked and the enzymes in the food are killed. What value do the nutrients in your foods or supplements have if they can't reach inside the cell? Liquid copals assist in delivering the nutrients inside the cells.

Pollution and poor nutrition cause the cell to form a shell around itself to protect it from the toxic environment. This thickened cell wall prevents nutrients from entering the cell. The copals may be the best delivery system known because they have the ability to penetrate the thickened cell wall and carry nutrients inside. It is always a good idea to have the liquid copals in your mineral and enzyme supplements. Healthy cells lead to a healthy body!

EMOTIONS
All the liquid copals seem to work on the emotions. You never know what smell will trigger an emotion for someone. When I first smelled a liquid copal blend containing Spruce, Cinnamon and Orange, I burst into tears. I had no control over my emotions. I couldn't stop the tears from coming. It felt as if a heavy feeling of hurt was being sucked out of me, leaving me in peace. The smell brought back some buried emotions I thought were gone years earlier. Now when I smell that same blend it is just beautiful. The emotion behind it was released and I was allowed to heal. That is how fast an emotional

healing can take place with the liquid copals. We call it the "breathe and blow" method. You breathe in the oil through your nose and blow out the emotion through your mouth. For more information see the Emotional Training Workbook and DVD.

Some of the best oils to use for Emotional Work are:

Confidence	Guardian	Utopia
Grateful	Balance	Clarity
Magnify	Love	Baby Soft
Ylang Ylang	Geranium	Break Thru
DNA Repair	Rose	Dreamtime
Lavender	Passion for Life	
Faith	Present Moments	
Peacemaker		
Hormone Balance		

Medical scientists have found our bodies are biochemical machines. We can change the composition of our body by what we think and feel. What we think and believe to be true about our world, we manifest in our bodies. "Fear based emotions" cause crystals to form around the cells and in the tissues. These crystals prevent oxygen from getting to various parts of the body resulting in discomfort and disease. When these crystals are eliminated, oxygen can then restore health to the body.

When we carry pain in our bodies, we need to look and see what adverse emotions we might be harboring. Every time we have an emotion, a chemical is created. Through the chemicals they create, emotions move from the circulatory system of the emotional body to the physical body where they actually alter the blood chemistry. This causes the physical body to express or suppress a feeling. Suppressing a feeling adds another layer to a previously formed crystal. The action of expressing the feeling returns the blood chemistry to normal.

82

When we suppress our fears or refuse to talk to the person with whom we are having a conflict, the chemicals in the blood collect somewhere in the body. Our failure to express our love may develop a problem in our heart as a result of blocked energy. Using essential oils has allowed many people to deal with their pent-up emotions quickly and effortlessly. When minerals are used along with the essential oils, they provide the most powerful and incredible tools we have discovered for healing the body, mind and spirit.

ENDOCRINE

Anise Seed	Basil	Cinnamon Bark
Chamomile	Clary Sage	Clove Bud
Melaleuca	Nutmeg	Sage
Spearmint	Coriander	Cypress
Spruce	Rose	Myrtle
Frankincense	Jasmine	Geranium
Helichrysum	Myrrh	Patchouli
Juniper Berry	Lavender	Marjoram
Black Cumin	Peppermint	Thyme
Holy Basil	Black Pepper	Vitality

The Endocrine System is the glands of the body. They produce substances called hormones that are secreted into the blood. These hormones act to regulate, integrate and coordinate a wide variety of chemical processes carried out by the other tissues and organs of the body.

The thyroid gland is located at the base of the neck. The hormones produced by the thyroid affect the general level of acidity of all the cells in the body. The thyroid acts much like a thermostat might, only on a chemical level. Iodine is a specific mineral for the thyroid. Zinc and copper also help support it. Foods that contain iodine are seafood, kelp, eggs, papayas, mango, pineapple and dulse. The adrenal glands are located above each kidney. Essential oils that may be beneficial for the adrenal cortex are: Vitality, Nutmeg, Sage and Geranium.

Widely distributed through the substance of the pancreas are small collections of cells called Pancreatic Islets. This is where the hormone insulin is produced. (Enzymes have been known to help inflammatory diseases of the pancreas.) Insulin is one of the main hormones that regulate the metabolism of sugar in the body and control the amount of sugar in the blood. The oils and minerals for the pancreas are selenium, chromium, vanadium, Coriander, Cypress, Helichrysum and Vitality. Stevia extract and Nature's Nutrients have been used to assist in stabilizing the sugar level. Holy Basil has been used in treating Type II diabetes.

The ovaries in the female and the testes in the male are also endocrine glands, producing hormones that regulate sexual development and reproduction. The essential oils of Fennel, Clary Sage, Geranium, Sage, Ylang Ylang, Bergamot and Yarrow have been very effective in overcoming many of the problems related to the reproductive organs. The progesterone cream Ebion Living sells contains the essential oils and has been found to be beneficial in supporting the reproductive organs.

IMMUNE / LYMPH

IMMUNE:

Clary Sage	Cinnamon	Melaleuca
Bergamot	Coriander	Lemon
Tea Tree	Black Cumin	Eucalyptus
Frankincense	Thyme	Myrrh
Rosemary	Rose	Lavender
Mt. Savory	Rosewood	Spruce
Oregano	Fortify	Freedom Plus
Spice Traders	Exodus	

LYMPHATIC - (all the organs in Immune System)

Cypress	Grapefruit	Helichrysum
Lavender	Lemon	Lemongrass
Orange	Sage	Lime
Sandalwood	Tangerine	Freedom Plus

The immune system is made of specialized organs and cells. Under the overall supervision of the brain, the immune system is programmed to protect the body against foreign invaders. When the immune system is not functioning properly, the results can be serious illness or death. The five major things that may cause a weak immune system are stress, fatigue, diet, environment and drinking unpurified water.

When our resistance is "down," or we are exposed to a large number of disease organisms (antigens), we may become ill. Our immune system must be able to deal with the antigens with which it has had no previous contact. Although it has the capacity to recognize and produce antibodies against some one million to one billion specific antigens, the immune system can not foresee every possible antigen that might come along. Sooner or later, a new antigen will enter our body, and the immune system must be able to combat it.

During the first phase of infection, white blood cells attack the invaders at the site of infection, engulfing the antigens and breaking them apart. The first line of white cells is then followed by a second line of white cells removing them from the site of infection, to eliminate the toxins or other harmful substances. During this battle, the blood supply to the digestive system is reduced (which is why we lose our appetite) and our temperature rises (we call it a fever). These changes are necessary to speed up the chemical reaction required for our recovery. So much intense energy is expanded on the visible cellular level that little energy is left for muscular action. The reason we cannot think too clearly during this phase of the battle is the brain is confused by poisons in the blood, resulting from the destroyed invaders as well as the elevated temperature.

When the infection is controlled, the macrophages return to the lymphoid tissue,

carrying with them particles of the destroyed antigen. Future defense cells result from these macrophages. Since these cells contain portions of the invaders, a later infection by the same invaders is immediately recognized and stopped.

Once our body has been exposed to a particular antigen and survived the attack, our immune system has a "memory" of that antigen. This long-term memory is an important feature of immune functioning. We may not be exposed to the same antigen for years after the first attack, but whenever we encounter that antigen again, our immune system will be ready for it and the antigen will be rapidly removed.

In his book, Practice of Aromatherapy, Dr. Jean Valnet, says, "Antibiotics act by modifying the chemical constitution of the microbes, so that the antibodies the organism produces for its own defense will be effective only against a modified germ. To put it plainly, the cure of an illness by means of antibiotics is a chancy business, less reliable in fact than natural recovery itself, which leaves the patient strengthened against any new infection."

The white cells differ according to their function. In the immune system the main fighting troops are the Neutrophils, B cells, T cells and Macrophages. Their job is to circulate through the blood, locate, trap and destroy threatening invaders. Both B and T cells begin their existence in the liver of a nine-week old fetus. They then migrate to the bone marrow, where they begin to follow different lines of development, specializing into varying kinds of "stem" or precursor cells.

The T cells then migrate from the bone marrow to the thymus gland, while the B cells remain in the bone marrow. The B cells are bone marrow-derived and the T cells are thymus-derived. The B and T cells also have distinct methods of dealing with antigens. Basically, if the invader is a bacterium, the B cells are responsible. The T cells are responsible for defending against fungi, parasites, and those viruses that attack from within the body's cells.

Neutrophils and Macrophages are called into play once an antigen has been recognized. They have the function of gobbling up antigens. The lymphatic system is the commander and the Neutrophils, Macrophages, B cells and T cells are somewhat akin to combat troops. The brain is, however, the center of all decision making and can be made to control aspects of immune functioning, even the lymph cells.

The lymphatic system is another name for all the organs of the immune system. It is comprised of two subdivisions: primary and secondary organs. The primary organs of immunity are the thymus and bone marrow. The secondary organs include the lymph nodes, spleen, tonsils, appendix, Peyer's patches and small-specialized lymph nodules in the membranes of the intestines. The fighting cells of immunity are produced in the primary organs but do not actually come into contact with foreign invaders until they reach the secondary organs where they initiate their defensive response.

The Lymphatic System is a network of small vessels, resembling blood vessels, by which lymph circulates throughout the body carrying food from the blood to the cells, picking up fats from the small intestines, and carrying body wastes to the blood. The tissues of the body, which comprise bones, flesh, and organs, excrete waste products as a result of their work. These must be quickly removed, or the tissues involved will suffer damage. The cleansing process of the body is performed by the lymphatic system. The most important function of the lymphatic system is to keep the blood proteins circulating. Other than that, they drain

away the lymph that has lost its nutrients by feeding the cells. This "dead fluid," along with the dead cells and poisonous waste that have been produced as a result of cell work, must be continually drained away. At rest, the lymph system will drain away about I.2 - 2.0 ml. of "dead fluid" per minute. During activity it can drain away about 20 ml. of "dead fluid" per minute.

The lymph is filled with waste products that pass through the lymph nodes. The lymph nodes fulfill the function of filter beds. These nodes form secretions and possess cells that have the power to neutralize, dissolve, destroy or take up the debris or waste products that may be in the body.

The liver plays a large role in detoxifying the body. After the lymph system neutralizes or dissolves the toxic wastes and renders the poisons inert, the lymph that is returned into the veins will be in a state of comparative purity. If the lymph system fails to function properly, it can cause hepatitis, infection of the liver and every other "itis" you can think of.

Even though the lymph system acts like a modern sewage treatment facility, it is literally the tree of life inside the body. When this system fails to function properly, excess blood proteins along with excess fluid and poisons build up in the body and pain, loss of energy, infection and disease take place.

Keep in mind that any mental, emotional, or muscular activity puts cells to work, and working cells put off poisons that must be carried off by the lymph system. When the lymphatic system does not work well, the resulting condition is called congestion. Congestion is a form of lymphatic stagnation.

When lymphatic stagnation takes place through cells not having access to the elimination organs such as the skin, bronchial tubes, throat, and digestive tract, the poisons build up in the lymph system. These poisons may begin to cause an oozing of the lymph through these open surfaces. This oozing is a common condition known as catarrh or inflammation of the mucous membranes of the nose and throat.

Tonsils, like all other lymphatic tissue, produce lymphocytes that protect the body from infection. Recurring tonsillitis calls for a good look at your Immune System. If the tonsils are swollen and inflamed, gargle with the essential oils of Lemon, Tea Tree, Clove Buds, Spice Traders, or Fortify. Surgical removal should be a last resort.

We say a person has a cold or cough when the lymphatic circulation of that part of the respiratory tract is so retarded that the lymph must be extruded through the lining surfaces of the tissues concerned. If this happens to the skin, it will produce sores or rashes. Eating foods that are of a cleansing nature, exercising, taking minerals, enzymes and essential oils may assist in restoring the lymph circulation to normal. The importance of the function of our lymphatic system in keeping the blood proteins circulating cannot be stressed too strongly. Loss of energy in your body is one of the first indications of a clogged lymph system.

MUSCULAR
ACHES & PAINS:

Birch	Lavender	Sport Pro
Helichrysum	Ginger	Basil
Marjoram	Nutmeg	Oregano
Freedom Plus	Peppermint	True Blue

FATIGUE:

Grapefruit	Holy Basil	Ravintsara

INFLAMMATION:

Sport Pro	Birch	Relief
Freedom Plus	Peppermint	Basil
Helichrysum	Elemi	Lavender

MUSCLES / NERVES:

Sports Pro	Basil	Helichrysum
Peppermint	Marjoram	Rosemary
True Blue	Nerve Repair	Soothing Relief

SPASMS:

Rosemary	Black Pepper	True Blue
Relief	Peppermint	Sport Pro

TONE:

Lemongrass	Toning	Fennel
Slim and Trim		

There are three types of muscles: 1) the voluntary muscles such as those that cover the skeletal framework; 2) the involuntary or smooth muscles such as those that control the movement of food through the digestive tract; and 3) the cardiac muscle which produces the contractions of the heart. Muscles, aside from their obvious power to enable us to move, also help maintain our posture and are responsible for a large part of our body heat.

Like bones, muscles enlarge and grow stronger when used regularly. The more you sit around, the more the muscle fiber becomes permeated by fat. In a majority of people, the muscles account for almost half their body weight. Much ill health and musculoskeletal degeneration may occur later in life because of our inability to relax. It may be important to learn to relax your muscles and thereby relax your whole body.

Emotional tensions may be translated into muscular contractions. Chronic muscle tension may be based on emotions that have been inwardly repressed instead of being outwardly expressed. Those suffering from disorders such as arthritis or muscular rheumatism may benefit from learning to relax. It may be that much of their problem is due to inner tension. Most musculoskeletal disorders may respond quickly to the oils. Some problems may be directly

86

attributable to tissue nutrition, lymph drainage, or over-relaxation or contraction of the muscles.

Use MSM, cleansing supplements, minerals and essential oils when there is a build up of toxins in the tissue. Drink plenty of water to ensure that waste materials are voided from the body.

NERVOUS

Basil	Cardamom	Nerve Repair
Cinnamon	Thyme	Clary Sage
Black Cumin	Birch	Frankincense
Helichrysum	Nutmeg	Lemongrass
Marjoram	Peppermint	Soothing Relief
Mt. Savory	Ravintsara	Sport Pro
Rose	Rosemary	Rosewood
Sage	Sandalwood	Spearmint
Spikenard	Spruce	Tangerine
Ylang Ylang	Relief	True Blue
Freedom Plus	Freedom	Focus
Circle of Life	DNA Repair	
Peaceful Moments		

The Nervous System thought of as the electrical wiring and control panel of the human body. The nerves are the wires that carry electrical signals from the sense organs (receptors) that are widely distributed inside as well as on the surface of the body. The nerves transmit these signals via a main trunk line and relay system, the spinal cord, to a central control panel and switchboard, the brain. In the brain, the signals are registered, analyzed, and interpreted. The brain sends out its order, also in the form of electrical impulses, through another set of nerves traveling via the same trunk line and relay system, spinal cord, to the muscles, organs, or glands of the body which must respond to the original stimulus.

There are two groups of sense organs (receptors): the General Sense Organs which are sensitive to touch, pain and temperature and the Special Sense Organs which include sight, taste, smell and hearing. The nerves that carry

the orders from the brain are also divided into two groups: The Motor Nerves that transmit impulses to the muscles and the Visceral Nerves that go to the glands and internal organs.

Anxiety may be a background cause of much ill health and is often in response to stress. Anxiety is described as "fear spread thin" and may call for oils that restore and relax the nervous system. Chamomile may assist in calming an over-stressed nervous system as well as Rose, Lavender, and Neroli. The essential oils may be used in a massage or diffused into the air.

Migraines are intense, usually one-sided, headaches sometimes signaled by a distortion of vision and often accompanied by nausea, vomiting, and sensitivity to light. Migraine sufferers are often high achievers and perfectionists who need to learn how to adapt a more relaxed lifestyle.

Minerals that work for migraines are magnesium and sulfur. Essential oils that will help are Migraine Relief, Freedom Plus, Focus, Serenity, True Blue, Soothing Relief, Peppermint and Marjoram. Some women experience migraines around the time of their period. In these cases, there is usually a hormonal imbalance and the use of a progesterone cream and minerals have been known to help.

Insomnia is most commonly a reflection of high levels of tension. Relaxation, regular exercise, and the oils of Lavender, Valerian Root, or Serenity applied on the temples and bottom of the feet will assist one to relax and sleep. Neuralgia nerve pains may often be caused by a lack of nutrients to the affected area. This is why so called "pain blockers" will not solve the problem. By using essential oils and minerals, it will assist in bringing the needed nutrients to the affected area.

RESPIRATORY

Basil	Cedarwood	Clove Bud
Cypress	Eucalyptus	Fir
Frankincense	Rosemary	Tea Tree
Helichrysum	Breathe EZ	Hyssop
Juniper Berry	Marjoram	Myrrh
Rejuvenate	Myrtle	Orange
Oregano	Peppermint	Spruce
Ravintsara	Rose	Sandalwood
Focus	Fortify	Thyme
Anise Seed	Black Cumin	Litsea Cubaba
Freedom Plus	Melaleuca	Mt. Savory
Resp EZ	Spice Trader	

UPPER RESPIRATORY:

Eucalyptus	Peppermint	Thyme
Ravintsara	Rosemary	Breathe EZ

BEST for DIFFUSING:

Breathe EZ	Rosemary	Ravintsara

We, like all other living creatures, need a constant supply of oxygen at the cell level. As we breathe, our respiratory system is perfectly designed to extract the oxygen from the air. While we can go without water and food for a few days, we perish within minutes without oxygen.

The function of the respiratory system is to bring air into contact with the blood. The oxygen in the air is absorbed into the blood. The carbon dioxide in the blood, which is a waste product of the body, is blown off. The blood coming from the heart and entering the lungs is rich in carbon dioxide and poor in oxygen. In the lungs, the carbon dioxide is removed from the blood and a fresh supply of oxygen is picked up. The blood, now rich in oxygen, is returned to the heart and then on to all parts of the body. Our lungs are important for elimination of waste products. Shallow breathing or smoking may put a strain on the lungs and other organs of elimination, such as the kidneys, bowels, skin and heart.

The over production of mucus may sometimes be a desperate attempt by the body to discharge waste material that has not been properly eliminated by the bowels, kidney and skin. To reduce mucus production, it may be essential to focus on diet. Also, hot lemon drinks may assist in the reduction of mucus production.

Suppressed emotional factors, like grief, may sometimes lead to blocked upper respiratory passages. Our lungs are connected to our emotions – just think about laughing or crying. If a person with asthma has difficulty in expressing feelings, it may be worth the effort to explore their feelings. For asthma, it may be wise to add minerals and oils that support the nervous system such as Chamomile or Soothing Relief. Deep breathing may also strengthen our connection with our feelings and, if practiced regularly, could assist asthma.

A virus that replicates inside the cells of the host may cause colds. Because of this, antibiotic drugs (which destroy bacteria outside cells) may not even touch a cold virus. This is where the minerals of silver and zinc go to work. Essential oils have the ability to penetrate the cell walls and thus may create an environment in which the virus cannot live. Viruses may also cause voice loss. Good oils to use would be Black Cumin, Oregano, Thyme, Fortify, and Spice Traders. Sinusitis, inflammation of the four air-containing cavities in the skull, usually occurs after a cold. The sinuses are lined with mucous membranes that react to infection by producing mucus to incapacitate infecting bacteria. Diffusing essential oils may be one of the most effective ways to treat upper-respiratory mucus and sinusitis. Dilute Oregano 50% in olive oil and take three drops, three times a day with meals. A sore throat may be effectively treated using essential oils. Gargle with warm water using a couple of drops of Clove Bud, Peppermint, Tea Tree, Lemon, or Spice Traders. Because oils are antibiotic, they are effective in knocking out infecting organisms and in loosening sticky mucus allowing the nasal and sinus passages to open.

Coughing is a reflex response to anything blocking the airways. The oils, which may help in decreasing coughing, are aimed at killing off bacteria, loosening and expelling mucus secretions and restoring lung function. Constant coughs and colds are also a warning to strengthen the immune system.

An affective way to treat a respiratory problem may be through the rectum. The nerves provide direct travel to the respiratory area. In a suppository application use the liquid copals along with carrier oil.

SKIN

Cedarwood	Chamomile	Elemi
Clary Sage	Bergamot	Cypress
Frankincense	Jasmine	Tea Tree
Baby Soft	Geranium	Vetiver
Helichrysum	Lavender	Juniper Berry
Patchouli	Lemongrass	Ylang Ylang
Myrrh	Petitgrain	Rosemary
Rose	Rosewood	Sandalwood
Cucumber	Renew	Skin Care
Balance		

The skin is an active and vital organ essential to our survival. The elastic nature of the skin is designed to guard the sensitive tissues and our organs against physical or chemical damage. The skin also prevents the loss of body fluids and regulates the body temperature.

An adult has several million sweat glands that fulfill many of the basic functions of the kidneys. The skin has sometimes been called the third kidney. If the kidneys fail to function properly, a heavier demand is made on the sweat glands. Conversely, should the sweat glands be

ineffective, an added burden falls on the kidneys. Sweat itself forms a protective acid mantle on the skin and helps kill harmful bacteria. Oils that induce sweating, such as Peppermint and Ginger, may be added to a hot bath to assist the body in ridding itself of toxic waste.

The skin is also a sense organ. It is made up of microscopic nerve endings that send information about temperature, touch, pressure, or pain to the brain. Our skin is a mirror of our general well being and treating skin diseases requires an overall evaluation of the sufferer's health. When the essential oils are unable to reach deep enough to achieve results, you may want to consider working from the inside out with minerals, enzymes, and Nature's Nutrients. It is the nature of skin to bring to the surface problems that would otherwise do damage at a deeper level.

A lady shared with me her use of the following essential oils for her skin cancer. In one teaspoon of carrier oil, she used two drops of Geranium, three drops of Frankincense and two drops of Cypress. She frequently applied these oils to her skin daily. This treatment yielded good results. To this blend I would add three drops of Cedarwood because of its beneficial effects on skin diseases.

Acne is chronic inflammation of the sebaceous gland. To control acne, the diet could consist mainly of fresh vegetables and fruits. Essential oils, minerals and MSM are beneficial to help clear up acne. You can also use the oils to assist in purifying the blood. Since acne is caused by blockage of the follicles by sebum, a steam bath using Rosemary may be beneficial in opening the pores. Consider using a spray bottle (see Acne).

Warts come from a virus that is mildly contagious and spread by contact. Oils that have been known to help when applied directly on the wart are Oregano, Thyme, Cinnamon, Lemon, Tea Tree, or Spice Traders. These oils are hot, be careful to only put it on the wart. If it gets on the skin, dilute with carrier oil.

Psoriasis is a relatively common skin disease. The pattern of psoriasis is over-activity of the external layer of the body. Many sufferers lead stressful lives, characterized by a restlessness and over-activity that is mirrored by their skin. In some cases, psoriasis first occurs after a bad shock. It would be important if you suffer from psoriasis to take definite measures to reduce stress by practicing regular exercise and relaxation techniques. The minerals, enzymes and Nature's Nutrients may also be beneficial. Use the essential oils of Chamomile, Lavender and Serenity to relax and strengthen the nervous system.

Psoriasis is usually more active in the winter months. External applications that can help the dryness of the skin are Baby Soft, Chamomile, and Sandalwood mixed in carrier oil. Avoid using soaps that dry the skin and lotions with mineral oil. Mineral oil is a by-product of gasoline and very drying to the skin.

When the skin constantly flakes off, substantial quantities of nutrients are lost. You may find it beneficial to replace these nutrients by increasing your Nature's Nutrients intake. Psoriatic skin contains abnormally high levels of cholesterol, according to the New York Journal of Medicine (II/15/80). You may want to add lecithin to your diet.

Eczema is a non-contagious inflammatory disease of the skin. The common house dust mite is frequently to blame. In a 2 oz spray bottle put 15 drops of Purify, fill with water, shake, spray around the room especially the carpets and mattresses, then vacuum. This should help control dust mites.

Eczema may also be caused by nutritional deficiencies. The enzymes, minerals, and Nature's Nutrients would again be beneficial to use. The skin will quickly return to normal once the deficiency is corrected. Remember, to have healthy skin you need to work both from the "outside / in" and from the "inside / out."

SKELETAL

Sport Pro	Birch	Clove Bud
Cedarwood	Fir	Cypress
Spruce	Sandalwood	Confidence
Ginger	Hyssop	Juniper Berry
Lemon	Peppermint	Relief
True Blue	Soothing Relief	

The Skeletal System is comprised of the bones and strong ligament bands that hold the bones together. The 206 bones which form the structural framework of the body also serve to protect and support the delicate internal organs of the body such as the brain, heart, and lungs. The skeleton is not a dead group of bones, but each bone is a live organ. The bones receive a rich supply of blood. Within the marrow cavities of the bone, the red and white blood cells are constantly being formed.

The spine supports both the trunk and head and also protects the spinal cord. You may be able to influence the organs of the body by working the oils along each side of the spine in the Vita Flex application. Use caution when doing this technique to avoid applying a lot of pressure or using hot oils.

With our modern diet, a complete range of vitamins and trace minerals may be necessary for bone and muscle repair. Nature's Nutrients is considered a food and contains them both. Bones are continually being renewed with the old bone being taken out and new bone being created so it is important to give your body the building blocks it needs.

90

URINARY

Cardamom	Cedarwood	Black Cumin
Freedom Plus	Clary Sage	Eucalyptus
Fennel	Rosemary	Vitality
Frankincense	Geranium	Grapefruit
Juniper Berry	Fortify	Lemongrass
Black Pepper	Sage	Sandalwood
Thyme	Spice Traders	

The Urinary System consists of the two kidneys and their ureters, the bladder, and urethra. The function of this system is to remove waste products from the blood and extract vital chemicals and body fluids from the waste products before returning them to the blood.

All the blood of the body passes through the kidneys over 500 times in the course of a day. The kidneys continually process this blood, carefully screening out those substances that are waste products and conserving those elements that must be retained. The kidneys are among the body's most important organs. Without their constant hard work, we would be poisoned by our own waste. The importance of the kidneys rests as much with what they reabsorb as with what is voided as urine. About 98% of the water and most of the nutrients are reabsorbed. Waste products such as urea, which is formed from the breakdown of protein, are passed into the urine and voided from the body.

Kidneys are responsible for controlling the acid/alkaline balance of the body. They are also able to monitor and raise the body's blood pressure by means of a hormone. High blood pressure may be a sign of an underlying kidney disorder. The kidneys also produce a substance that stimulates bone marrow to make red blood cells. The calcium and magnesium are good minerals to use for the kidneys.

Essential oils may be beneficial not only for urinary disorders, but also in assisting the body's cleansing as a whole. It is usually advisable to start by using diuretic copals such as Tangerine, Fennel, Patchouli, Sage, Juniper Berry and Grapefruit in a massage. These copals assist in strengthening the kidneys and encouraging them to excrete debris in the urine. Increase the amount of water you drink to give the kidneys a better chance to flush out toxins.

Cystitis is inflammation of the bladder and can occur at any age. It is about 20 times more common in women than men. Minerals and the essential oils of Basil, Lavender, Chamomile, and Peppermint will fight the inflammation.

The prostate gland is an accessory organ of the male reproductive system. The gland is normally about the size of a chestnut, but if it becomes inflamed or enlarged, it may exert pressure on the urethra or it may block the outlet to the bladder obstructing the flow of urine. If this happens, it can cause:

- An interrupted or difficult urination (so called dribbling incontinence)
- Urgent urination
- Frequent urination - especially at night
- Potential pain associated with urination

Urine trapped in the bladder may become infected and cause cystitis. In addition, the backward pressure can lead to kidney infection. The high level of urea retained in the blood may sometimes be a cause of mental confusion.

91

NUTRITIONAL TIPS & INFORMATION
This section covers a lot of things I am interest in and would like to share.

In recent history, mankind has managed to drastically change the chemistry of the environment in which we live. Chemicals are released into the soil, water, and air affecting all aspects of our life causing free radicals. Every individual living in an industrialized nation, whether they are living in the mountains or a rural area, is bombarded daily by over 10,000 free radical hits. If you work around paints, chemicals, computers or other electronic devices, your exposure is still greater. Under optimum conditions, the body can deal with the free radicals that occur during its natural processes. Because of the ever-increasing prevalence of free radicals in the environment, the body's ability to fight back is overtaxed.

Poor quality diets and refined food combined with extensive use of antibiotics in medicine and agriculture may cause many of us to experience a kind of "internal" pollution. There is a reason why some people go through life content and happy, with hardly a digestive worry and others have to put up with the constant, nagging "background noise" of an unhappy stomach. The reason is too many "bad" bacteria and not enough good bacteria – healthy flora – in your gut.

When you feel bloated, gassy, cramped, or just uncomfortable after meals, it's usually because you have exceeded your body's ability to digest your food. Excess gas can form when you don't have enough good bacteria (probiotics) and enzymes to break down food quickly and painlessly in your small intestine. The undigested food passes to your large intestine where bad, gas-producing bacteria feast on these scraps and give off carbon dioxide, hydrogen and methane gas as a byproduct.

Internal pollution occurs when unhealthful bacteria overcome the healthful bacteria in the intestinal tract. When the gas gets trapped, you get that full, bloated feeling and as it builds us you feel as if you are being stabbed. This is where a good probiotic is needed. When you have enough of the "good guys" gas is dramatically reduced

PROBIOTICS PLUS:
Probiotics can have a far-reaching impact on your health. They provide protection in a toxic world and assist in restoring the internal balance that not only protects against illness but promotes optimal health and vitality. Many people are unaware that daily exposure to our environment and even some habits considered healthy – like taking antibiotics, drinking chlorinated water and using antibacterial soap – often kill these good bacteria essential for health. Supplementing with probiotics is an effective, safe and easy way to incorporate them into your daily life.

Unless you are living in an absolutely pure environment, you are being exposed to bad bacteria constantly. It is important to understand that bacteria are everywhere, but do not be too worried because you have been living with them since you were a baby. It is up to you to keep your friendly bacteria healthy and assist them in outnumbering the bad. When there is a "bacterial imbalance" you can struggle with symptoms, such as fatigue, for weeks or months before an ideal balance has been re-established. Probiotics fulfill very specific tasks that are critical to your overall health. Here are some examples of what probiotics the good bacteria can do:

- Bifidobacteria produce important B vitamins, including niacin, B6, folic acid and biotin and when there is fewer Bifidobacteria may dramatically affect the body's production of these B vitamins – the anti-stress vitamins.
- Probiotics manufacture the enzyme lactase which helps us digest dairy products; improves digestive efficiency and encourage proper bowel function – literally recycling toxins.
- Works to reduce cholesterol levels by contributing to cholesterol metabolism and

utilization.

- Stimulate a positive, powerful immune system response throughout the body.
- Probiotics can assist in treating illnesses.

The following are some of the key reasons for "bacterial imbalance":

- Antibiotic use - One of the most common ways we disrupt intestinal bacterial balance is through the use of antibiotics.
- Estrogen use - Birth control pills and prescription estrogen have been shown to disrupt normal intestinal flora balance.
- Travel - Any kind, especially out of the country, can influence the condition of the digestive tract.
- Stress - Emotional and physical stress can cause bacterial imbalance.
- Lifestyle factors - Lack of physical activity, not drinking enough fresh water, low-fiber diet, stress, negative attitude, smoking and drinking alcohol will most likely result in digestive disharmony.
- Food and water-borne contaminants - Four of the most common causes of food-borne infections are salmonella, staphylococcus, E. coli and listeria. One of the first lines of defense against these pathogens is your internal microflora.

One negative by-product of antibiotic overuse is the over-growth of Candida. Fortunately, Candida responds very favorably to probiotics treatment. It is important when you take antibiotics that you also take probiotics. Take your probiotics supplement during or right after a meal. Then take your antibiotic at a different time during the day.

Taking the probiotics with the evening meal may be best so the good bacteria have at least eight hours to colonize before you take your antibiotic again. Probiotics should also be used in conjunction with antifungal prescriptions to help preserve, enhance and replenish good bacteria. It is always a good idea to take probiotics when traveling or if you experience a bad reaction to something you ate or drank. It is certainly in your best interest to keep your good bacteria in abundance and your digestive system stocked with them. The friendly bacteria continuously die off and are eliminated from the body. It is vital to continually replenish your supply of good bacteria to offset the bad bacteria that make their way into your system via food, air, water, and our environment.

It is suggested you supplement with probiotics if you have a family history of cancer, heart disease or digestive problems (including lactose intolerance); you are over the age of 55; are taking antibiotics; travel frequently; have high cholesterol; are under emotional and/or physical stress; frequently experience constipation or diarrhea; and are inactive and have an unhealthy diet. The scientific community has confirmed you need at least 1 billion living cells in your probiotics supplement. The best probiotics are those that are stable at room temperature making them convenient to take along when traveling.

The essential oils are another healing modality that has been known for thousands of years for its ability to benefit the body and support health. There is evidence to support the fact that essential oils fight microbes, fungus, bacteria, viruses, parasites, and inflammation to mention a few of their benefits.

The major benefits of using oils are their ability to deliver nutrients to our nutritionally depleted cells. The oils act as the delivery system to send the nutrients directly into the cell and through the compromised cell wall, which has had the pH altered due to chemical toxins in the body. The oils assist our immune system to fight off diseases allowing our body to rebuild and regain its healthy condition. It is important to remember that when all the cells in your body are healthy, then you will be healthy.

AGELESS PLUS:

It stands without question that if the immune system is strengthened, numerous ailments and illnesses can be aided and alleviated. The ingredients in "Ageless Plus" are enzyme active stabilized rice concentrates (Nature's Nutrients), organic Black Cumin oil, organically grown Muscadine Grape powder, wild Tsi-Ahga a Native American Sacred herb, and the heart of garlic Allicin-Release Product (ARP). Each one is demonstrated in scientific research to strengthen, support and modulate the immune response in different ways. When these ingredients are combined their singular efforts are synergized.

The Black Cumin has impressive scientific research which shows it to have very beneficial, anti-bacterial and anti-viral properties. Long used as a traditional remedy for colds and viral infections, Black Cumin is still a good choice to use against illness. In contrast to synthetic cold and flu medications, using "Ageless Plus" to overcome a cold can help strengthen the immune system so the body is able to heal quickly and resist additional infections. People who are under extreme stress tend to be much more susceptible to illness. The Black Cumin contains unsaturated fatty acids, linoleic acid and gamma Linolenic - all essential for a healthy immune system.

One of the most important components in Black Cumin is the volatile oil Nigellone which is known to be effective for bronchial asthma and respiratory allergies. It has the ability to expand and relax the airways, reduces the release of histamines into the bloodstream and works against allergic reactions. It has been shown that allergic symptoms are reduced up to 90% with long-term supplementation with Black Cumin. The saponin and nigellin in Black Cumin give it its appetite-enhancing and digestion-stimulating qualities. It acts as an antihistamine and pain reliever.

Research on Black Cumin has focused on its positive effects on the immune system. Scientists know that Black Cumin stimulates bone marrow and immune cells, raises the interferon production, protects the body against viruses, destroys tumor cells and inhibits infection. Research revealed that Black Cumin possesses antibiotic properties that act against a wide spectrum of gram-positive and gram-negative bacteria. In side-by-side tests Black Cumin matched or exceeded the ampicillin's effectiveness in defeating gram-positive bacteria.

Laboratory tests also indicate that Black Cumin may hold promise in fighting cancer cells. The study shows that Black Cumin is superior to other medicines in many regards. It proved to be more effective than chemotherapy and radiation treatments - without their serious side effects. The Cancer Immuno-Biology Laboratory of South Carolina ran a series of experiments in which mice were infected with tumor cells. Two thirds of the animals treated with Black Cumin oil were still alive thirty days after being infected. In contrast, **all** the mice that did not receive Black Cumin treatment died within the same time period.

Concentration problems are not limited to the elderly. The main causes are lack of oxygen and nutrients to the brain, stress, pressure and internal conflicts that lower the ability to concentrate. Using Black Cumin regularly may ensure you will keep a clear head even in old age.

Muscadine Grape and Seeds, another ingredient in Ageless Plus, contains resveratrol which is known to be anti-aging. Researchers believe the evidence is sufficiently strong to conclude that a single dose of resveratrol is able to induce beneficial physiologic responses. It contains higher levels of antioxidants which protect and restore immune function resulting in a wide variety of protection throughout the body.

Garlic, the next ingredient in Ageless Plus, has been used successfully for thousands of years for a wide variety of conditions. Garlic has established itself as a successful food/medicine, and now scientists agree that the allicin in garlic is the key to the majority of garlic's success. The chemistry of garlic is extremely complex and even though allicin was discovered in 1944, there are very few supplements or garlic-based products that contain any allicin, let alone 100% pure absorbable allicin. Some proven activities of allicin are:

- Reduces blood pressure
- Kills microscopic organisms
- Kills poisonous bacteria, parasites and fungal infections
- Reduces high blood cholesterol
- Removes lead, mercury and other toxic materials
- Reduces or prevents cancer tumors
- Removes dangerous free radicals
- Repairs the immune system
- Delays aging
- Keeps blood circulation healthy thereby reducing blood fibrinogen

In the past year drug stores, supermarkets and mass merchandisers in the United States have sold more than 5 million units of garlic. This makes garlic the most popular herbal product according to Information Resources, Inc., and yet none of those consumers are getting what they actually need (the Allicin) from the garlic product. With the new patented extraction method for stabilizing Allicin, the Ageless Plus can offer the product people thought they were buying.

Here is a variety of conditions that the allicin formulation will assist as mentioned in the book Allicin the Heart of Garlic: acne, AIDS, animal bites, arthritis, asthma, bad breath, bacterial infections, bladder infections, blood pressure, boils, Candida, canker sores, cholesterol control, circulation, cold sores, colds and flu, cough and respiratory infections, diabetes, diarrhea, delayed aging, eye infections, Ebola and Dengue fever, eczema, hay fever, gingivitis, head lice, hepatitis, heavy metal

contamination, impetigo, irritable bowel syndrome, MRSA infections, parasites, peptic ulcer, psoriasis, SARS, scabies, shingles, sinusitis, sore throat, tuberculosis, warts and wound healing.

The Story of Tsi-Ahga: The Nez Perce Indians of the Upper Plateau region of the Pacific Northwest were expert observers of animals. In the winter, the Nez Perce observed that the elk, moose and deer often dug down through the snow around stumps or fallen trees and ate the hard fungi that grew on them. These animals, more often than not, quickly recovered from their weakened and ill state and successfully survived the harsh mountain winters. The Nez Perce, believing that the Sky Father and the Earth Mother had given them a gift, made this woody fungus one of their most important medicines and placed it at the center of the Medicine Wheel. In the center of the wheel, Tsi-Ahga became synonymous with the defense and protection provided by the Creator. It was added to the pemmican, the staple diet of the Nez Perce.

As a consequence, where other tribes suffered from the diseases the trappers and traders passed on to them, the Nez Perce People did not. In fact, when the Lewis and Clark expedition passed through their territory, and even stayed with them, there was no outbreak of disease consequent to their visit even though the expedition journal mentioned many of the party suffered from measles just as they were passing through the region. Clark himself was one of the sufferers.

Tsi-Ahga is derived from Conks that grow on certain cone-bearing trees. The 3-beta-D-glucans which make up part of the cellular structure of these Conks cause a pan-systemic modulation of T-Cells, Macrophages and Neutrophil White Blood Cells, when ingested. In fact, it has been established that the number and viability of these particular cells is increased by as much as 4000% within 20 hours after taking Tsi-Ahga! Macrophages and Neutrophils are the two cells upon which all other

95

Immune Cells depend. You can have many viable B-Cells and T-Cells, but they will not be effective without the programming provided by these "Communicator" cells. Tsi-Ahga also contains bitter triterpene compounds that support the thymus and spleen (essential to insuring that immune cells are properly programmed), anti-tumor polysaccharides, blood pressure-reducing angiotensin re-uptake inhibitors and perhaps the highest source of germanium in nature. Germanium is an oxygen catalyst and one of the most powerful free-radical scavengers found in nature.

I felt the following research by Phillip R. (Cloudpiler) Landis very interesting and should be made available. It helps us better understand how beneficial the Ageless Plus is and may be the very thing your family needs to survive a flu outbreak.

Avian Flu Research Abstract

Date: June 2006 - Sept. 2006
Introduction: Avian Influenza is a common problem for poultry operations in the United States. Most commercial poultry plants are under continuous quarantine because of the very real threat of the introduction of new and mutable strains of Influenza.

The Battery Method of commercial poultry production provides the perfect laboratory to study virus mutability, since the environment is not only not natural (requiring the virus to change is modus operendi), but also the close quarters and significantly diminished immune systems of the battery birds provides an excellent pathway for the "skipping of generations." In other words, what might have taken countless generations to create in the wild is dramatically facilitated by the Battery Method.

Research Description: A small backyard flock of squabbling pigeons was used for this research. The pigeons were housed in a facility with less than one square foot floor space per bird, with nest boxes attached to the back wall. This population density exceeds that of most Battery Production Facilities and so goes further in concentrating the transmissibility and mutability of virus.

Control Group: Ten birds were housed separately but with the same approximate living quarters. These were used as controls.

The Test Group: The test group consisted of twenty six birds housed as described above. The Test Group was fed a ration containing "Ageless Plus" mixed into the feed for one week prior to the test. The Control Group was fed normally.

Two Infected Pigeons: these pigeons were obtained from a local, wild flock. The birds were demonstrating the classic symptoms of Avian Influenza. One infected bird was placed in each of the pens and the groups were observed for seven days.

Control Group: All of the control birds were infected with the Influenza within three days of exposure. All of the control group birds, including the original vector, died within the seven days of the observation period.

Test Group: Although all of the test group birds demonstrated symptoms of infection, i.e., nasal discharge, coughing, swollen eyes, etc., none of the twenty six test birds died during the observation period. The only bird in the test pen to succumb was the original vector.

Follow up: The Test Group continued to receive Ageless Plus and were observed for three months post-infection. During that time, only two birds died – one of egg binding and another became entangled in the mesh wiring of the pen. None of the birds exhibited any symptoms after the initial bout of flu. The hens all went off production and did not become eggy again until the following spring. Molt was as usual.

96

Postscript: It is interesting to note that, after the research was terminated, and the test group birds were no longer receiving Ageless Plus in their feed, the loft was infected by a different wild strain of Influenza which had been transported to the loft by wild infection and two thirds of the birds died within the first five days after infection. Those that survived never returned to normal production.

Findings: The commercial product "Ageless Plus" provided the immune support needed for the closely quartered birds to fight Influenza. The results of the Test Group were not unlike an influenza epidemic that is "winding down." Individuals became symptomatic but were able to fight off the virus. The results of the Control Group were reminiscent of the first weeks of an epidemic, when the virus is the most dangerous. These observations are compelling and demonstrate a need for greater research into the effects of Beta1;3, 1;6 glucan use in prevention of Influenza Outbreak.

Cloudpiler's own story – "When I was told that I had only weeks to live and that there was nothing that could be done, you might imagine that I was devastated. My complete confidence had always been in the miracle of modern medicine. But that miracle was not to be available to me.

Despairing, I sought advice from a man I had met many years earlier while undertaking a vision quest among my people, the Nez Perce Indians of Northeastern Idaho. He told me to take the wood fungus known as "Tsi-Ahga" and keep a piece of it in my mouth at all times. Up to receiving this suggestion, I had been losing copious amounts of blood from the bowel as the disease literally ate me up from the inside. I was dying.

So, even though I must admit I had always considered the wood fungi to be at best unsafe and at worst downright poisonous, what did I have to lose? I did what I was told and a miracle happened. Within just a few short weeks the bleeding stopped and within a year my disease was in complete remission. Now, the disease that was killing me and had engulfed my entire G.I. tract is almost completely gone. The gift of the Earth Mother has given me back my life."

~~~~~~~~~~

E. T. of Indiana writes: "I just have to tell you that I am so excited and pleased since the first capsule of Ageless Plus that I took. My blood pressure has dropped from 148 / 64 to 125 / 54 and my brain fog cleared in a very short time! My breathing is even improved--- breathing deeper, with a feeling of wellness that I thought was long gone! I thank God for who formulated this wonderful product and for the person who made sure that I tried it."

T. W. from Utah writes: "I had a virus and for three months it left me with an earache that was very painful and miserable. It felt like an inner ear infection or block. I had a little bit of temporary relief once when we went on a trip and in the higher elevations my ear popped. I took one of your Ageless Plus capsules at night and the next morning I took another one. When came to work I announced that my ear was clear. I could hear again! I was so thrilled I could not believe it."

"I have also had a ringing in the ear for years and the ringing has just quit...it went away. I feel this has all been sinus related and I am so grateful to you for such a wonderful product. I also have experienced more energy. I now have my energy back and I am not a couch potato at night. I have a ruptured disc in my back and I am starting to do things I have not been able to do for years. I have only used 1/2 a bottle so far and it has been just great. I can't thank you enough for this great product."

Just this morning my daughter told me how bad her allergies get when she gets busy and goes without her Ageless Plus for three days. She can feel the difference when she takes the Ageless Plus regularly.

VITAMIN C PLUS:

I have always suggested you take vitamin C with your Ageless Plus since the Tsi-Ahga seems to be more effective when your intake of vitamin C is adequate. In my search for a good vitamin C I noticed about 95% of them were poorly absorbed and full of fillers such as cellulose, silica or dextrose. I have found a vitamin C that contains Calcium Ascorbate, Bioflavinoids, Alfalfa, Parsley, Rutin, Hesperidin and no fillers.

Vitamin C is vital for tissue growth and repair, the formation of teeth and bones, wound healing, and resistance to infections. Vitamin C plays a part in almost all aspects of our health and well-being. This powerful vitamin also contributes to the production of stress hormones and the neurotransmitter serotonin which enhances your mood. Vitamin C may help prevent arteriosclerosis by combating abnormal blood clotting, high blood pressure and plaque buildup leading to hardening of the arteries. Because vitamin C is an antioxidant which battles damage-causing free radicals, it may also help to prevent cancer. Recently, scientific evidence has indicated that the vitamin works along with vitamin E in this role: The synergism of the two vitamins produces a greater effect than either vitamin can separately.

As an antioxidant, vitamin C scavenges free radicals in the body and protects tissues from oxidative stress. It promotes the absorption of iron, while preventing its oxidation and is a vital co-factor to the formation of collagen, the connective tissue that supports arterial walls, skin, bones and teeth. More vitamin C is contained in the adrenal glands than any other organ in the body and is required at higher levels during times of stress. Physical stresses on the body such as ingestion of heavy metals, cigarette smoking, infections, extreme temperatures and chronic use of certain medications such as aspirin also signal the need for increased intake of vitamin C.

The human body cannot manufacture vitamin C. We need to get it from food and supplements. Vitamin C is a "water soluble" vitamin which means that it "washes out" of the body every day. Yesterday's excess vitamin C is gone today! After 10 to 20 days your vitamin C is totally gone in the absence of further ingestion. It is a major anti-oxidant in the body and needs to be replaced daily. The richest natural sources of vitamin C are fruits and vegetables. Good sources are: oranges, honeydew melon, strawberries, cantaloupe, mangoes, kiwifruit, watermelon, papaya, grapefruit, broccoli, tomatoes, cauliflower, cabbage and citrus juices. Raw and cooked leafy greens (turnip greens, kale, spinach), red and green peppers, potatoes, winter squash, raspberries, blueberries, cranberries and pineapple.

Vitamin C is absorbed by the intestines. The presence of large quantities of sugar either in the intestines or in the blood can slow absorption. Once ingested, vitamin C is readily absorbed by the intestines and continues through the watery components tissues that make up the human body and is said to uphold the body's natural equilibrium.

Many people think they are doing very well when they take 500 milligrams, or even 1,000 milligrams of vitamin C. Since vitamin C is so beneficial everyone ought to be taking much larger doses. The actual amount of vitamin C that will be used in the body depends on the health or sickness of the body. The body, in some cases, can absorb as much as 50,000 mg. The minimum daily requirement of vitamin C now being recommended was based on keeping a person from getting scurvy and not health.

Now that you know you do need vitamin C every day, the question is how much do you need? Well, you can have a sudden demand placed on the body where several thousand milligrams of vitamin C might be "used up" in just a few hours. Or, you may go through several very calm days, no stress and not need more than a small amount of vitamin C each of those days. Just know, if you are under stress it would be a good time for you to take more vitamin C. Some people believe that when your urine is yellow you are probably excreting an excess of vitamin C that was taken.

Another way to check on your vitamin C is to look at your fingernails. If the little white half moons can been seen on **all** your nails you have adequate Vitamin C at the time. It will disappear from the little fingers first. Vitamin C is surely one of the cheapest forms of health insurance there is. What you should worry about is when and if your urine is NOT yellow and the white moons are gone from your fingernails. That might mean that ALL the vitamin C you are taking has been used up and that, perhaps, you should even take MORE!

EATING HABITS:
It is also very important to eat a good diet with plenty of fresh fruits and vegetables, whole grains, nuts and seeds. Avoid eating excess fat, refined sugar, and foods high in additives and preservatives. Eat moderate levels of protein (approximately 15% to 20% of your calories) and fat (approximately 20% of your calories), while increasing levels of complex carbohydrates (approximately 60% of your calories). Substitute organically raised animals and organically grown fruits and vegetables whenever possible. Drink plenty of purified water. A home water purification system is very important.

Use foods that contain the complete vitamin B complex such as the Nature's Nutrients. It has been found that the B-complex vitamins take care of 96% of the deficiencies in the body. They are water-soluble and any excess is not stored in the body; they must be replaced daily. It is important to remember that all B-vitamins should be taken together because they are interrelated in function. You may take additional doses of an individual B vitamin over a short period of time, but do not take massive doses for extended periods. Here is a story that helps understand the importance of eating right:

"FARMER THOMAS PARR OUT LIVED NINE MONARCHS AND DIED AT AGE 152."
Englishman Thomas Parr was a farmer - most of his life. Nevertheless, he's buried in Westminster Abbey alongside kings, queens, poets and other noble dead. Today, you can still see his small headstone imbedded in the wall of that massive church. Why did he merit this exalted burial? Well, his claim to fame is that several documents prove he truly lived for 152 years.

When the church investigated, the parish register in his native village claimed he was baptized in 1483. Legal records state that he inherited his father's small farm in 1518. A marriage document proves he took a wife in 1563, at age eighty. Another marriage certificate attests that he married a second time in 1605 at the age of 122.

In September 1635, he gained the attention of King Charles I who invited Parr to the palace for a visit. Parr's quick wit, matchless memory and endless stories made him a peerless entertainer. The King was so amused that he bid Parr to reside in the palace. Parr cheerfully accepted and sold his farm.

Of course, he stopped eating his simple country food, and continued amusing His Majesty while stuffing himself with the rich royal food. And in the middle of one of those meals only a few weeks after his arrival at the palace, Farmer Parr dropped dead at the age of 152. Fascinated by Parr's great age, Charles I instructed his surgeon, William Harvey, to perform an autopsy to discover what finally killed Parr. This surgeon's death certificate, still preserved in Latin, states that "acute indigestion brought on by indulgence in unaccustomed luxuries" was the cause of Parr's death. The rich food and wine of royalty proved too much for Farmer Parr.

Americans are dying from the same foods that killed Parr! Aren't we Americans consuming food that only royalty and the very rich could afford in Parr's day? Don't we eat large quantities of beef, chicken, pork and lamb loaded with animal fats? Don't we gobble down all kinds of cookies, cakes, pastries and other snacks? Farmer Parr outlived 9 kings and queens until he started eating their rich food!

Too many Americans have become candidates for heart disease, cancer, diabetes, arthritis and other diet related ailments. The people who recognize this danger have returned to eating natural foods, whole grains, unrefined oils, fresh vegetables, fruits and small amounts of fish and meat. These are the foods that Thomas Parr consumed most of his life.

NATURE'S NUTRIENTS:
Nature's Nutrients is one of the most nutrient-dense food sources on the planet. It is a whole food that is full of complex nutrients which work together synergistically to restore optimal health. Nature's Nutrients is the result of a specialized processing of rice concentrates and extracts. It consists of perfect chains of essential fatty acids, trace minerals, amino acids, PhytoNutrients, glyconutrients and over 90 powerful antioxidants including tocotrienols, which have been found to be 6,000 times more effective than vitamin E. Because they are in perfect ration, they are absorbed into the body – not as bits and pieces but as whole organic structures.

These structures repair different organ systems (like the heart and liver) on the cellular level. Its nutrients slow aging and aid the body to repair rebuild and restore. Its powerful glyconutrients help all nutrients we ingest to work better. The product is yeast-free, starch free and sugar-free. Because Nature's Nutrients is a food instead of a drug or supplement, there's no danger of overdosing on antioxidants or its other substances.

Natural antioxidants seldom work by themselves but are very effective as part of an antioxidant system in which there is synergistic action. Antioxidants protect our body from free radicals. The free radicals burn holes into the outer cell walls, depleting oxygen and damaging the DNA within.

The damage can lead to cell dysfunction, cell death, or worse – the transformation of the injured cells into cancerous cells. As a result of free radicals each one of the billions of cells in our body gets approximately 10,000 oxidative hits per day. This demonstrates why the consumption of potent antioxidants is crucial for our health.

The principal antioxidant compounds present in Nature's Nutrients are tocotrienols, tocopherols and oryzanols. The first two compounds include eight different chemical forms that together are commonly referred to as vitamin E. The least active tocotrienol antioxidant is 40 to 60 times more potent than vitamin E. The most active tocotrienol is up to 1,000 times that of vitamin E's alpha tocopherol. Furthermore, some of the compounds in Nature's Nutrients have over 10-times greater antioxidant activity than pycnogenol.

Nature's Nutrients contains the universal antioxidant lipoic acid. Lipoic acid is not only the ideal anti-aging antioxidant but also an essential coenzyme factor in the production of energy. Lipoic acid can go anywhere in the body because it's unique characteristic of being both water-and fat-soluble. Lipoic acid is good for diabetics since it stabilizes blood sugar to calm down sugar cravings and energy swings.

Glutathione is another antioxidant found in Nature's Nutrients. Glutathione helps in preventing and battling weight gain, hyperactivity, alcohol, sugar, caffeine addiction, allergies, arthritis, cataracts and lung, skin, prostate and bladder cancers. Half of the individuals over age 65 are deficient in glutathione which makes them susceptible to all kinds of disease, especially cancer. Glutathione acts as a detoxifier.

Nature's Nutrients contains the anti-aging antioxidant mineral selenium. Working together with vitamin E, it strengthens our immune system and thyroid functions and keeps our heart, liver and pancreas healthy. One of the surprises of selenium is its ability to fight cancer.

Another nutrient found in Nature's Nutrients is gamma-oryzanol which can be effective in reducing stress and lowering elevated cholesterol and triglyceride levels. Several studies show that gamma-oryzanol has beneficial effects on menopausal problems, hormone imbalances, head and neck injuries and other autonomic nervous system problems. For athletes, the gamma-oryzanol and ferulic acid combination found naturally in Nature's Nutrients has been shown to lead not only to increased muscle mass but also to improved strength, body composition, decrease in body fat, enhanced recovery times and less muscle soreness.

The Russian athletes found that vitamin B-15 (pangamic acid) increased oxygen to the cells, thus increasing the athletes' endurance, Nature's Nutrients is an excellent source of all the B Vitamins. If you are not eating nutrient-dense whole food, then you are not protecting or feeding your cells. Starving unprotected cells equals discomfort, disease, premature aging and death. Again, free radicals are the cause of virtually all disease.

Nature's Nutrients is a cell-ready food and the most nutrient-dense food source known. It not only contains one of the largest arrays of antioxidants, it also includes phytochemicals, vitamins, minerals, essential amino acids and the essential fatty acids. If it weren't for the fact that Nature's Nutrients is missing a few minerals, it would be the perfect food. With the essential fatty acids (oils of life) in Nature's Nutrients you have the mortar to hold your body together, protect the cells, improve hormone production and balance (insufficiency can cause P.M.S., menopausal problems, low testosterone and infertility), reduce brain fog, pain, UV damage to the skin and wrinkles. Essential fatty acids also protect against pesticides and other toxins.

Nature's Nutrients may offer protection from

premature aging, heart disease, osteoporosis, cancer, stroke, diabetes, arthritis, Alzheimer's disease and certain eye disease such as macular degeneration and cataracts. It provides the nutritional therapy and protection that our diet often doesn't have. This benefit is critical for individuals who experience fatigue and low energy and often turn to coffee, colas or other stimulants. Here's where Nature's Nutrients can be so helpful-- it gives natural support so there's no need for stimulants of any kind. The most dramatic results have been with diabetics and older people. Elderly people need the nutrients it offers. As a "natural" whole food, Nature's Nutrients gives the body what it needs.

Nature's Nutrients is having a profound effect on all kinds of people – from those with debilitating diseases to those who want to bring their health to a higher level. Nutrition is the key and Nature's Nutrients is the whole food that contains a symphony of nutrients. In combination, these nutrients can do much more than any single nutrient can do. As smart as we are, we still can't recreate in a pill what God has given to us naturally.

"When you implement an optimal nutrition program, don't expect rapid results because the body needs time to grow new improved cells," says Dr. Michael Colgan. After many years in sports nutrition, he feels the shortest program given any athlete is six months. It takes your body 3-6 months to completely replace its entire blood supply with healthier cells – incorporating the added nutrients – and a year to replace all its bones. Therefore, you need to make a commitment to stay on the Nature's Nutrients for at least six months.

If you are a parent, one the greatest gifts you can give your child is to start them on the Nature's Nutrients at a very young age. One way to save money is by eliminating from your pantry all products that are not whole foods and/or bio-available. You would spend over $200.00 on a multitude of products trying to get what Nature's Nutrients offers.

Basic Nature's Nutrients Bars are ones our family enjoys. One bar with 16 ounces of water is a complete meal. When kept individually wrapped in the fridge or freezer, they are ready to go in seconds. There are so many ways to vary the taste of this bar. I like to change the taste by adding drops of the Lemon, Lime, Nutmeg, Cinnamon or Orange essential oils to a batch of the bars. Just be creative, use your imagination and create the type of Nature's Nutrients Bars you will enjoy eating.

NATURE'S NUTRIENTS BARS - Mix together in a large bowl:
1 container of Nature's Nutrients (1#)
2 cups sesame seeds
1 ½ cups raisins
4 cups old fashion rolled oats (not instant)
1½ cups other chopped fruit of choice (papaya, apricots, pineapple, coconut, etc.)
2 ½ cups chopped nuts and sunflower seeds

In a sauce pan melt over low heat:
1 ½ cups sweetener (honey, maple syrup); 3 cups natural peanut butter or other nut butter; 1½ cups water. Pour over the dry mixture and shape into balls or bars. Wrap and put in fridge or freezer.

Guaranteed specifications in Nature's Nutrients:
Protein 12 – 16%; Fat 18 – 23%; Total Dietary Fiber 23 – 35%; Total Carbohydrates 45 – 55%

ENZYMES PLUS:
The importance of enzymes has long been ignored but now their involvement in daily body functions is becoming a major issue. The enzymatic content we have in our bodies is directly related to the quality of our health. Enzymes are needed for every chemical action and reaction in the body. They are an important factor for longevity, vitality, superior health, overcoming sickness and weight management. Without enzymes life cannot exist. Metabolic enzymes run all our organs, tissues, and cells. Minerals, vitamins and hormones need enzymes present to perform their work properly. They are the work force of the body. The better we maintain and build our enzyme reserves, the healthier we will be.

It is important to understand that enzymes initiate all cellular activity. Enzymes break down toxic substances so the body can eliminate them without damaging the elimination organs. Our immune system, bloodstream, liver, kidneys, spleen, pancreas, as well as our ability to see, think and breathe all depend upon enzymes. As we become enzyme deficient, we start to age faster.

A shortage of enzymes may cause serious health problems. Because enzymes must break down every food we eat into simpler building blocks, eating only cooked foods can eventually cause enzyme exhaustion at the cellular level. A human being is not maintained by his food intake, but rather, by what is digested. Cellular enzyme exhaustion lays the foundation for a weak immune system and ultimately disease. A common misconception is that vitamin and mineral supplements will make up for dietary deficiencies.

It is important to remember that without enzymes, nothing works in the body no matter how well formulated the supplement might be. If food is not completely digested, the body does not get the nutrients it needs. That is why people with food allergies often have vitamin and mineral deficiencies.

Enzymes ingested either in the form of raw, whole organic foods or supplements optimize digestion. Not only can allergies disappear but so can the accompanying vitamin and mineral deficiency as well. Vitamin and mineral deficiencies develop in a relatively short period of time-60 to 90 days-but enzyme deficiencies take longer to develop, simply because the body has so many compensation mechanisms. When an allergic reaction occurs, an enzyme deficiency has likely existed for months or even years prior to its onset.

Enzymes help to increase oxygen levels while helping to raise your pH. This can protect you from free radical damage. Plant enzymes provide energy directly to the individual cells and enhance the electromagnetic fields in the body causing increased energy. It is important to have an enzyme reserve for your body to draw from to maintain health. There are two ways to build the body's enzyme reserve: (1) by eating raw foods (especially papaya) and (2) by taking an enzyme supplement. Here are some of the ways we use up our enzyme reserve:

- During an illness or when under stress – enzymes are used up more rapidly.
- Athletes – any time the body temperature is raised enzymes are used up quickly.
- Over-eating cooked foods - causes the digestive organs to quickly use enzyme reserves. All foods, in their natural state, have an abundance of enzymes. However, as foods are heated past 118 degrees all enzymes are destroyed. This means the enzymes in all foods that are canned, baked, pasteurized, roasted, stewed, fried or microwaved are completely destroyed.
- Breaking down antigens - all diseases are considered to be systemic problems in natural therapeutics. The white blood cells help to destroy antigens and other toxins by engulfing them and digesting or partially destroying their substance making it easier for the body to eliminate. In most cases, they do this by secreting enzymes that break down the antigens so the body can eliminate them via the lymphatic system.
- Digest protein/release antigens - most antigens, bacteria, viruses and yeast are protein.

The digestion of protein is done by enzymes, not only in the digestive tract but also in the deposits in the bloodstream itself. Bacteria, yeast, antigens and other toxins enter the body through the digestive tract. If the immune system is not strong and healthy enough to destroy them, they attach onto food substances we eat and then multiply within the body. Substances causing allergies can also enter the body simply through the air we breathe. Antigens that cause allergies attach themselves to proteins in the blood and become deposited in the walls of tiny capillaries. The antigens then secrete substances that cause inflammations that result in swelling, hay fever, sneezing, hives and asthma.

Eat raw fruits and vegetables between meals helps to increase the enzyme activity through the whole body. It is important to realize that yeast is also a protein and can be digested by enzymes if the body has a constant and proper supply. The importance of understanding why undigested proteins, bacteria, and yeast enter the blood through the intestinal wall and have a toxic effect on our system cannot be stressed strongly enough. If the immune system is weakened, Candida Albicans, which live naturally in the intestinal tract and vaginal areas of human beings, can take over our whole body. Providing a continuous source of enzymes may eliminate yeast and most antigens (being protein).

Other ways to assist the enzymes in your body is to use the lemon copal to help keep the lymphatic system clean. Also provide a good probiotic and trace minerals. Minerals are important for enzyme functions. Zinc, for example, is part of every living cell and is essential for the activity of over 200 biological enzymes.

Cleansing and short fasts are beneficial because enzymes go to work to clean up undigested materials in the blood and to purify the entire body. They help digest toxic waste and gases thus helping to retard the aging process. They influence the thyroid gland and are a key to permanent weight loss. Enzymes can help dissolve cholesterol in the liver and other body parts, thereby controlling weight, which also protects your heart. They create a penetrating action on stored fats, dissolving them out of the body's adipose (fat) cells.

The importance of enzymes cannot be over emphasized. Nature's way of preserving the life force in cereal grains, legumes, tree nuts and seeds are by enzyme inhibitors. It was discovered in the 1940's that it is necessary to remove the enzyme inhibitors from our plant foods for proper digestion. The addition of supplemental enzymes will inactivate these inhibitors and enhance enzyme activity. Cooking will also destroy these inhibitors, but the enzymes will be destroyed as well. Another way we can accomplish the same goal is by sprouting. These enzyme rich foods lay dormant until activated by water. As the enzymes come to life, they inactivate the inhibitors and begin to sprout.

Research with laboratory animals indicates specific harmful effects from ingesting inhibitors. They include gastrointestinal problems, an extremely enlarged pancreas, excretion of large quantities of wasted enzymes and a condition of overall poor health. The total loss of pancreatic enzymes will lead to death. It is most important to soak or sprout your nuts, seeds, grains and beans, eat them with supplemental enzymes or cook them to avoid the harmful effects of enzyme inhibitors. The nuts, seeds, grains and beans require at least 24 hours of germination to totally dissipate enzyme inhibitors.

It's important to note that the digestibility of sprouted foods is unsurpassed because of their high quality and content of available enzymes. Tests have indicated that other nutrients in sprouts can increase from 50 to 400% when germinated. For example, millet and wheat contain over five times the amount of vitamin C when sprouted. Also, sprouts increase their original protein content during the germination process. The Vitamin B content also grows substantially with germination. These pre-digested foods rich in activated enzymes enhance the body's own internal enzyme activity. These food enzymes are present to help break down protein, fats and starches. It is more beneficial to eat cooked foods without enzymes than raw foods with them. The following foods are especially nourishing and

building for body tissue: almonds, apples, apricots, arrowroot, artichokes, barley, beets, carob, carrots, cayenne, cloves, comfrey, dandelion leaves, dates, fennel, figs, horseradish, lentils, mangos, oats, olive oil, prunes, pumpkin seeds, red clover, brown rice, sage, sesame seeds, sprouts, sweet potatoes, and watercress.

To take a lot of stress off the body while you build your enzyme reserves, you may choose to use an enzyme supplementation. Nothing can happen without enzymes. Nutrients that are present in the foods you eat cannot be utilized without enzymes. The work force of the body is in enzymes. Enzymes are important in meeting the demands of modern life-styles. What we put in our mouths strongly determines the daily and long-term quality of our lives. Improper eating habits are a major cause of our skyrocketing health-care costs today. We must learn to take control of our own health. If you want superior health and vitality, getting an adequate intake of enzymes will make the difference.

STEVIA:
The Stevia leaf is one of the most effective health restoring plants on earth. What Stevia does both inside the human body and on the skin is incredible. The following are some of the benefits of Stevia:

- *Sweeter than sugar:* Enjoy Stevia by itself or as a sweet liquid for cooking and baking. It has been used as a sweetener in Paraguay for over 1500 years and in surrounding countries for centuries. Stevia has a unique taste. In some poor grades of Stevia this taste may be accompanied by a bitter taste as well.
- *No calories:* Users can enjoy the benefits as a dietary supplement because it contains no calories.
- *Effectively regulates blood sugar:* Scientific research has revealed that Stevia effectively regulates either high or low blood sugar. An important benefit for

hypoglycemic individuals is that Stevia provides a rapid increase in energy levels and an increase in mental acuity.

- **Lowers blood pressure:** Studies have shown Stevia lowers elevated blood pressure without affecting normal blood pressure.
- **Inhibits bacteria and infectious organism growth:** Users of Stevia report a lower incidence of colds and flu. Also, when used as a mouthwash or added to toothpaste, Stevia inhibits the growth and reproduction of bacteria and other infectious organisms that cause tooth decay and gum disease.
- **Weight management aid:** Stevia contains no calories. Research indicates it significantly increases glucose tolerance and inhibits glucose absorption.
- **Curbs the sweet tooth:** People who use Stevia regularly have reported a decrease in their desire for sweets and fatty foods.
- **Digestion aid:** Stevia used on a daily basis improves digestion and gastrointestinal function. Stevia can soothe an upset stomach and help speed recovery from minor illnesses.
- **Curbs desire for Tobacco & Alcohol:** An interesting but undocumented claim made by many users is that drinking Stevia water reduces the desire for tobacco and alcoholic beverages.
- **Skin care (acne, wrinkles, seborrhea, dermatitis, and eczema):** Apply Stevia as a facial mask. Allow to dry at least 30-60 minutes. As it dries, you will feel the facial skin tightening. It effectively softens the skin and smoothes out wrinkles while helping to heal various skin blemishes including acne. It is easily washed away with warm water. A drop of Stevia may be applied directly on the blemish or on lip sores. Stevia may be highly effective when used on seborrhea, dermatitis and eczema.
- **Healing of cuts, wounds, blemishes and sores:** People report that a few drops of Stevia extract placed in cuts and wounds assist rapid healing without scarring. This will sting for several seconds followed by a significant lowering of pain.
- **For Flavor:** Sprinkle lightly over cereals, salads or cooked vegetables, enhancing their natural flavor.

Stevia is a wonderful plant that is currently used as a healthy, no-calorie sweetener, and the leaves are a nutritious food. Stevia is great for smoothing wrinkles, softening and beautifying the skin, healing blemishes and sores.

METHYL SULFONYL METHANE - MSM:

It is important you avoid confusing the good MSM for the poisonous MSG which is discuss later. In his book, The MSM Miracle, Earl L. Mindell explains how an organic form of sulfur has shown important therapeutic value in arthritis, diabetes, allergy, wound healing, eye problems, cramps, stress and even snoring. I recommend you read this book.

As our bodies age, our immune systems become increasingly compromised. Our tissues suffer higher levels of free radical damage which is accumulative. This can result in a wide range of age-related degenerative conditions and can make us more vulnerable to infectious diseases. MSM is a sulfur-carrying compound that magnifies the nutritional effect of vitamins and helps build the amino acids responsible for protein building and muscle formation. It supports the immune system and almost every major body function.

Some possible signs of sulfur deficiency are poor nail and hair growth, eczema, dermatitis, poor muscle tone, allergies, rheumatism, arthritis, weakening of the nervous system, constipation, gout, lowered libido, impairment of mental faculties, and Candida. Sulfur helps maintain the pH balance of the body, benefits insulin production, expels parasites, normalizes heart function, and excretes toxins from the liver. The following are some excerpts from the original patent documents on the benefits of MSM:

- **BODY:** Resistance to sun and wind burn. Benefits for eye inflammation. Oral Hygiene for mouth and gums and improved sense of taste and smell. Benefits internal organs and lung tissue providing relief from the symptoms of lung dysfunction. Speeds wound healing. Beneficial for allergies and other sensitivities, it controls problems associated with gastric hyper acidity, and relieves chronic constipation. MSM reduces or eliminates hypersensitivity problems associated with oral medications such as non-steroidal anti-arthritic agents. It provides relief from pain, stiffness and reduces swelling and inflammation. Enhancing the immune system, reduces hypertension, and is a mood elevator.
- **SKIN:** Beneficial for skin, internal organs, connective tissue, and dermatological disorders. MSM counteracts cross-linking of collagen associated with aging, improves adverse skin conditions, and has a favorable response in treating acne.
- **HAIR & NAILS:** It is beneficial for the scalp and improves hair and nail growth.
- **PAIN RELIEF:** Relieves acute pain, post-athletic activity fatigue, muscle and leg cramps, arthritis and other sources of pain.
- **DERMATOLOGICAL DISORDERS:** Acne (including Grade 4), acne Rosaceae, and other diverse dermatological problems which are often allergy related respond favorably to using MSM.
- **MUSCLE CRAMPS:** It has the ability to reduce or eliminate entirely muscle cramps, leg and back cramps after long periods of inactivity, or in athletes such as runners, football, basketball, and soccer players who experience cramps during the participation of their sport.

- **MENTAL NORMALCY:** Individuals on MSM generally reported increased alertness, reduced mood changes and very infrequent depression. A few patients on medication intermittently for depression observed that MSM relieved depression within hours rather than days as had been their prior experience with anti-depression medication.
- **PAIN ASSOCIATED WITH SYSTEMIC INFLAMMATORY DISORDERS:** Individuals with signs and symptoms of pain and inflammation associated with various musculoskeletal system disorders reported substantial and long lasting relief while including MSM in their daily diet. Migraine sufferers have obtained substantial relief with MSM.
- **PARASITIC INFECTIONS:** MSM has an alleviating effect on a variety of parasitic infections returning the parasite susceptible tissue to normalcy with no impairment or injury to the host.

The body uses MSM to create new, good healthy cells. Vitamins and amino acids work with MSM during this process. Without proper levels of MSM, our bodies are unable to build good healthy cells which leads to illness. Our body produces new cells 24 hours a day. If our body doesn't receive the proper nutrition and building materials it needs from the foods we eat, it will produce bad, dysfunctional cells. If we want a good flexible cell capable of maintaining good health, we need to eat foods that contain sulfur or supplement our diets with MSM.

MSM is a natural form of organic sulfur found in all living organisms. It is found in all foods – vegetables, fruits, meat, and milk. It is quickly lost from food when it is processed, cooked, and stored. The second you pick fruits or vegetables they rapidly begin losing their MSM. Even in meats, MSM is not as abundant as it used to be. Today animals are fed foods deficient in MSM.

When your body uses the MSM molecule to produce a new cell, the MSM is lost forever. We need to continuously replace the body's needed supply of MSM to produce new, healthy cells. Most normal diets do not supply the minimum requirement of MSM. It is absent in synthetic food additives, dietary mineral compositions, food substitutes and most fillers used to dilute or modify foods. With today's modern diet of processed foods, most diets are deficient in this important ingredient.

You will find MSM is as safe as drinking pure water. Because of its inert nature, MSM is non-allergenic and has no interfering or undesirable effects. It is estimated that the body uses up about 1/8 teaspoon of MSM each day, it uses what it needs, and the excess is flushed out. MSM is a free radical and foreign protein scavenger. It cleans the bloodstream so allergies to food and pollens go away in about three to four days. The body will use MSM wherever it is needed in your system. To maintain good healthy cells, you may find it beneficial to use MSM as a supplement in the morning and evening.

I found this information on Sulfur from The Natural Pharmacy, by Miriam Polunin and Christopher Robbins. "SULFUR: Used in medicine for at least 4,000 years. This was long before it was known that every cell in the human body contains sulfur, as do all plants and animal cells. In man, the mineral is concentrated in hair, nails and skin. May be used for scabies, acne, dandruff, skin problems, laxative, mild antiseptic, lower back pain, body odor, kidney, constipation, impotence, diarrhea, over sweating, lack of stamina and over sensitivity to the cold."

By now you've probably decided that MSM is something that would benefit you. How do we take this marvelous product? I must tell you it has what I call "an acquired taste." I have tried it several ways and will probably try several more until I find the way I can take it regularly. At first I put it in a glass of water, but that was too bitter. Next, I put it in my mouth and washed it down with water or juice. This

seems to work the best for me. I know the benefits well out-weigh the bitter taste. Make a promise to yourself not to go a day without your MSM.

HORMONAL BALANCE--ESTROGEN And PROGESTERONE:

When we talk about hormonal balance, we are talking about the relationship between the body's estrogen and natural progesterone levels. Many women and men lack sufficient progesterone levels due to a buildup of petrol-chemicals in the body, which significantly reduces the production of progesterone.

Stress, processed foods, and other problems unique to our society cause us to not get enough of the necessary nutrients to create a balance. If the systems responsible for creating balance do not get the progesterone they need, then they will try to steal it from other parts of the body. The result is everything from PMS, cramps, mood swings, and even the eventual deterioration of the bones called Osteoporosis. It is very important for a woman that is estrogen dominant to get her progesterone stores built up so her body can begin to create that critical balance.

Usually estrogen and progesterone have an antagonistic relationship with each other. High estrogen levels during the first half of a woman's cycle trigger the storage of water, sodium, fiber and other nutrients to prepare her body to support another life. Then progesterone levels go up in the last half of her cycle. If no pregnancy occurs, her body stops the manufacture of hormones. It is this sudden stop in the production of progesterone that causes the shedding of the endometrium lining (menses). The progesterone is almost totally created by the ovary but only in the months that women ovulate. So if a woman does not ovulate during a month, for whatever reason, then she will not create the progesterone needed to cause the flushing out, and this repeated storing without cleansing causes estrogen dominant symptoms.

The estrogen and progesterone in a woman work to balance each other. What the estrogen puts in, the progesterone takes out. Here are some balances:

ESTROGEN
Creates proliferate endometrium
Reduces oxygen levels in all cells
Decreases Libido
Impairs blood sugar control
Interferes with thyroid hormone
Increases bodies fat
Depression and headaches
Increased risk of breast cancer

PROGESTERONE
Maintains secretary endometrium
Restores proper cell oxygen levels
Restores Libido
Normalizes blood sugar levels
Facilitates thyroid hormone action
Help use fat for energy
Natural anti-depressant
Helps prevent breast cancer

When the two hormones are in balance, a woman goes from cycle to cycle with no problems. It is only when a woman gets out of balance that problems occur. Women have receptor sites in their bodies that the progesterone cleans off so the estrogen can work. The estrogen then clears off the receptor sites for the progesterone. Since a woman can make more estrogen than progesterone, she may have a hormonal imbalance most of her life.

In the February 1997 issue, of Life Enhancement magazine, Jonathan Wright, MD said, "We need to take the last 40 years worth of study on so-called 'estrogen,' jam it in the waste basket and start over. All of those studies involved giving human beings horse estrogen. The next time I see a menopausal horse, I will be happy to prescribe Premarin, a horse estrogen! But for menopausal people, we need people hormones."

From the same article Dr. John Lee, MD said his research revealed the use of natural progesterone had been studied as far back as the 1930's, when it was first synthesized from the fats and oils of certain plants. Conventional medicine abandoned it in the '50s and '60s when the pharmaceutical companies discovered they couldn't patent natural progesterone, so they created chemical substitutes for progesterone that had some progesterone-like activity. These substitutes were used in birth control pills and blocked real progesterone from working. He said, "It is money and control. Since natural progesterone is sold over the counter, doctors lose control, and no one can make much money on it because it can't be patented."

When taking progesterone it is important to use a natural source. Synthetic sources of progesterone can cause even more problems than they solve. Natural progesterone is found in over 5,000 foods, but by the time the foods reach us after processing, there is very little left for our bodies to use. This is one reason why so many women and men are progesterone deficient.

Dr. Lee has stated that the best way to take natural progesterone into the body is apply it topically. He shared his concern regarding the delivery agents of most of the progesterone and/or yam creams on the market that use chemicals as their delivery agent. A good progesterone cream contains natural progesterone along with the best natural topical delivery agent available on the market – essential oils. When oils are added to the cream, the body is able to recognize it as food and then carry the nutrients into the cells.

From Dr. Lee's research, and from reports of people using progesterone cream, the following is a partial list of ailments favorably effected by using progesterone cream:

Wrinkles   Sinusitis
Digestion   Bloating

Improved libido Improved bone density
Hot flashes Depression
PMS Acne
Inflammatory diseases Hair loss
Prostate problems Fat being used for energy
Excess alcohol Normalized blood clotting
Breast tenderness Insomnia
Improved Weight loss Cold extremities
Bruise easily Lactation
Asthma Infertility
Joint pain Toxemia of pregnancy
Swelling Backache
Spontaneous abortion Water retention
Exhaustion Breast engorgement
Mood swings Sore throat
Fibromyalgia Frustration
Herpes simplex (#1) Improves brain function
Reduction of fibroid growth
Proper cell oxygen levels restored
Normalized blood sugar levels
Normalized zinc and copper levels
Protection against breast cancer
Improved thyroid hormone action
Helps with headaches and migraines

Dr. Lee says in most cases women having difficulty losing weight usually have too much estrogen and not enough progesterone in the body. He also indicates any excess progesterone will be converted to estrogen if the body is lacking estrogen. A natural progesterone cream with essential oils may be a good way to get some of your much needed progesterone. Since every person is different, it is important to determine the amount and times you use progesterone cream. Some people use it two times a day, some only once a day and others will use it every other day. As you use the progesterone cream you should be able to tell the amount that feels best for you. Start out slowly and build up.

THE ACID ALKALINE BODY BALANCE:

We have an acid/alkaline balance in our bodies. If this balance is not kept in the right proportion, illness will occur. All foods, elements, and compounds have different pH levels. If the pH is between 0 – 6.9 it is acid 7 is neutral and from 7.1 – 14 is an alkaline pH. Vinegar, for instance, is a fruit acid with a pH of around 2.5 and is known as an acidic solution. Calcium, on the other hand, has a pH of 12 and is known as an alkaline element. The foods we eat and our lifestyle has an overall effect on the pH of our body, even anger changes our pH.

Certain parts of the body, including the center of each cell, are alkaline by function and are supposed to be in the pH range of about 7.2. The outside medium of each cell is acidic by function and should be in the pH range of 4. The body is designed to maintain these two distinct pH levels. The body is electric. The difference between these two pH levels provides for electrical frequency functions within the cell. These ranges determine how much energy you have and also the clarity of thought and emotional balance.

Both pH levels must stay in their respective ranges, out of the middle area, for wellness to be realized. In other words, your upper pH must stay high, (about 6.8 to 7.4) and your lower pH must stay low (about 2.5). As you go through an average stressful day and eat acid foods, the pH levels move toward each other. If this is continued over a period of time, you enter the middle danger zone. Your resistance will go down and you will be susceptible to various internal parasites and invading bacteria. Viruses and many other diseases begin to prey upon your body when your pH is out of balance. As you get sicker and sicker, the difference between the pH levels moves closer and closer together. When both levels meet it is called death because the needed electrical frequency call 'life force' is no longer generated.

When the blood loses its alkalinity and starts to become more acidic, the foundation of health is undermined. Many authorities believe disease develops due to a lowering of the function and resistance of the body because of chronic acidosis.

This creates an environment where we become vulnerable to runaway yeast and fungus overgrowth. Preserving this alkalinity (pH balance) is the bedrock on which sound health and strong bodies are built. Dr. George W. Crile, past head of the Crile Clinic in Cleveland said, "There is no natural death. All deaths from so-called natural causes are merely the end-point of a progressive acid saturation." Acidosis precedes and provokes disease.

Cells adapt to an acidic condition by mutating and becoming malignant. Long-term acidic conditions in our bodies provide perfect environments for cancer and auto-immune diseases. Most people with these fatal diseases also have Candida which results from the fluids being out of balance.

Yeast infection is caused by a group of yeast like fungi called Candida. Candida is the most common, but it's not the only one. Everyone has a certain amount of Candida living on and in them, but not everyone develops Candida. Yeast lives on moist areas of the body such as the lining of the mouth and the vagina. Yeast has become more of a problem in recent years because several modern drugs such as antibiotics, steroids, and birth control pills throw the body's pH out of balance causing yeast overgrowth. The essential oils that have been helpful for keeping in Candida in check including Bergamot, Black Cumin, Clary Sage, Eucalyptus, Tea Tree, Mountain Savory, Myrrh, Patchouli, Rosemary, Rosewood, Spearmint, and Spruce. There is no better essential oil than Frankincense to boost the immune system. It is important to stay away from sugar products (commercial foods) that feed the yeast.

The naturally occurring yeast and fungi in the body thrive in an acid terrain. To help you understand this, an acidic solution is to fungi what oxygen is to man. These same yeast and fungi are responsible for secreting a large number of poisons called mycotoxins which are believed to be one of the root causes of many diseases and debilitating conditions.

Many cancers have been linked to mycotoxins. For example, the fungus Aspergillus flavus, which infests stored peanuts, not only generates cancer in laboratory animals but has been documented as the prime culprit in many liver cancers in humans.

Illness occurs when our bodies are too toxic and therefore too acidic. All infections, viruses, bacteria, parasites, and cancers are anaerobic and die in the upper pH level of 6.9 or the lower range outside the cell. They simply cannot breathe in these conditions and therefore cannot live. Understanding how to balance our internal chemistry holds a secret to success in healing and restoring the acid/alkaline pH balance. The optimal pH for bodily fluids is slightly alkaline. By balancing the body's pH and creating a more alkaline environment, you choke off the production of diseases-producing mycotoxins. With pH balance restored, the body can regain vigor and health.

Refined commercial foods are acid foods. Acid foods are addictive. They cause over-eating and weight problems. Whole natural foods have a balanced pH. The best way to inhibit yeast and fungus overgrowth in the body is by adhering to a diet without many of the acid forming foods such as meats, dairy products, flour, grains, and sugars. Unfortunately, this is a tough task for many of us. Most people don't have the determination to overcome their bad eating habits! You won't get a simpler solution for returning to health than that of eating whole, live food. Using a good plant based enzyme that contains essential oils will also assist you as you use the whole live foods. It will take time before you reverse the effects of many years of eating commercially processed foods.

It would be impossible to eat everything raw. Whenever you cook your vegetables, lightly steam them. Avoid using any processed canned vegetables and fruits. They will sustain life but because they are dead food they will never build health. Live people need live, alkaline, raw foods.

Symptoms associated with acidosis include: frequent sighing, insomnia, water retention, recessed eyes, rheumatoid arthritis, migraine headaches, dry hard stools, abnormally low blood pressure, difficulty swallowing, burning in the mouth and/or under the tongue, sensitivity of teeth to vinegar and acidic fruits, bumps on the tongue or the roof of the mouth, foul-smelling stools accompanied by a burning sensation in the anus, and alternating constipation and diarrhea.

When your body is acidic it will try to return you to an alkaline state by calling on your stored reserves of alkaline minerals: sodium, calcium, potassium and magnesium. If you continue eating foods that are highly acid forming, you leach even more alkaline minerals from your body creating a mineral deficiency that becomes severe over time.

Some causes of acidosis include kidney, liver and adrenal disorders, improper diet, malnutrition, obesity, ketosis, anger, stress, fear, anorexia, toxemia, fever, and consumption of excessive amounts of niacin, vitamin C, or aspirin. Diabetics often suffer from acidosis. Stomach ulcers are often associated with this condition. Excess blood acidity weakens the respiratory system resulting in less oxygen available to the cells. This leads to further fatigue. Deep breathing and diffusing the liquid copals assists in getting more oxygen into the body. In an oxygen-rich internal environment, disease is unable to grow. Other signs of an acid condition are forgetfulness and constantly disorganized. A balanced body contributes to clear thinking and precise action.

Remember, an acidic body contains excess hydrogen which is harmful. In order for the body to balance the hydrogen it must combine with available oxygen to form water, a harmless compound, thereby neutralizing the excess hydrogen, and excreting it from the body. Have you ever wondered why you urinate frequently even though you haven't been drinking a lot of liquid? Could it be you are

acidic and the body is combining the extra harmful hydrogen with oxygen to rid it from the body? This results in a constant depletion of internal oxygen. Other necessary metabolic processes are unable to function properly without sufficient oxygen and this leads to degeneration, another reason to limit your intake of acid-forming foods.

Acidosis is often a contributing cause of drug addiction. The nicotine in tobacco and caffeine in coffee are alkaloids, or alkalizing substances, that neutralize acids in the body. Yet as a whole, tobacco and coffee are acid forming. As we become more acidic the more addicted we get to these alkaloids. Other examples of alkaloid containing substances are cocaine, marijuana, morphine, amphetamines and heroine. A properly balanced alkaline diet may assist in eliminating addictive behavior.

Alkalosis is a condition in which the body is too alkaline. It is less common than acidosis and produces over excitability of the nervous system. The symptoms may be manifested as a highly nervous condition, including hyperventilation, sore muscles, creaking joints, bursitis, drowsiness, protruding eyes, asthma, allergies, hypertension, hypothermia, edema, night cramps and coughs, chronic indigestion, vomiting, too-rapid blood clotting, thick blood, menstrual problems, hard dry stools, thickening of the skin, and even seizures. Alkalosis may cause calcium to build up in the body as in bone spurs.

Alkalosis is often the result of excessive intake of alkaline drugs such as sodium bicarbonate for the treatment of gastritis or peptic ulcers. It can also result from high cholesterol, excessive vomiting, endocrine imbalance, poor diet, diarrhea, and osteoarthritis. Working to get and keep your body in a proper pH balance will be one of the best things you can do for your health. By eating plenty of vegetables, fruits, nuts, seeds, sprouts, berries and herbs, we are actually assisting our bodies to get alkalizing minerals. Not getting enough vital nutrients causes acidosis, an increase in acidity in the body. In Dr. Baroody's book "Alkalize or Die," he states, "The countless names of illnesses do not really matter. What does matter is that they all come from the same root cause… too much tissue acid waste in the body!"

pH PLUS:

It was designed to reverse and regulate low pH for maintaining optimum alkalinity at the cellular level. With its high concentration of minerals, trace minerals and vitamins the pH Plus works to achieve a homeostatic balance of the body's chemistry. Every living cell on the planet, plant or animal, depend on minerals for their proper structure and function. The pH Plus contains many alkalizing properties as well as a full spectrum of ionic plant minerals needed by our bodies. The complete ingredients are as follows:

Organic Dandelion: Rich in vitamins and minerals A, B1, B2, B3, C, E, calcium, chromium, iron, magnesium, manganese, phosphorus, potassium, sodium, selenium, silicon, and zinc. The therapeutic properties of the dandelion helps to regulate blood sugar levels, cleanses the kidneys and liver, helps with allergies and skin conditions, is considered a diuretic, laxative, choleretic, tonic, antioxidant and is anti-inflammatory.

Organic Watercress: Contains beta-carotene and vitamins B1, B2, B6, C and E. It is high in minerals such as copper, calcium, phosphorus, magnesium, potassium and sodium. Watercress has antioxidant and anti-cancer properties, protects the eyes, helps maintain the skin, promotes healing of wounds, burns or tendons and promotes bone formation.

Elemental Magnesium: An essential mineral for more than 300 biochemical reactions in the body and assists the body's absorption of calcium. The health benefits of magnesium include the transmission of nerve impulses, body temperature regulation, detoxification, keeping the heart

healthy, regulating blood pressure, maintains muscle function and the formation of healthy bones and teeth. Magnesium is also good for backaches, migraines, insomnia, depression and diabetes.

Broken Cell Wall Chlorella: Has large amounts of chlorophyll, enzymes, vitamins B-complex, C, B-carotene, B1, B2, B6, B12 and K. It includes vitamins and minerals such as niacin, pantothenic acid, folic acid, biotin, choline, lipoic acid inositol, phosphorus, calcium, zinc, iodine, magnesium, iron and cooper. The therapeutic properties include stimulating the immune system to protect from infections and cancers, stimulates the production of interferon, tissue repair and the production of red blood cells, increases oxygen to the cells, brain, assists in digestion, cleanses the bloodstream, liver, kidneys and feeds the friendly flora in the bowels.

Wild Royal Jelly: High in vitamin B, A, C, D E and K, minerals, 18 amino acids and 15% Aspartic acid (α-amino acid). The therapeutic properties include accelerating healing, strengthening the immune system, is antibiotic and antiviral, lowers cholesterol, builds tissue and muscle and regenerates cells. Also beneficial for chronic fatigue, liver disease, kidney problems, insomnia, stomach ulcers, skin disorders nervous disorders and arthritis.

Ionic Crystaline Calcium: Despite all of the hype, coral calcium for the most part is harmful to the body. There is only a small percentage, less than 8%, of good, useful calcium found in coral calcium. A special process is used to extract ionized elemental calcium that maintains the aragonite crystalline structure. It takes 13 pounds of regular Ionized Coral Calcium to make 1 pound of this organic concentrate. This 13:1 extract is a very fine powder, only 3.3 microns in particle size. The size, structure, and ionization of the calcium concentrate enables better absorption and effective calcium assimilation. According to scientific studies by Dr. Yamauchi, this calcium concentrate is at least 6 times more soluble in water than that of calcium carbonate CaCO3. It also does not build up in the system causing bone spurs and heart valve problems, like most all other calcium supplements.

Organic Bio-available Sulfur: All cells need sulfur. It is beneficial for skin conditions, allergies, asthma, arthritis, emphysema, diabetics, kidney problems and high blood pressure.

Organic Turmeric: Rich in fiber, iron, manganese, potassium and vitamin B6. The therapeutic properties of turmeric include: detoxification of the liver, reducing inflammation and cholesterol levels, improves blood circulation, and encourages the growth of digestive flora.

Wild Native American Tsi-Ahga: The 3-beta-D-glucans, which make up part of the cellular structure of Tsi-Ahga, cause a pan-systemic modulation of T-Cells. Tsi-Ahga contains bitter triterpene compounds that support the thymus and spleen (essential to insuring that immune cells are properly programmed), anti-tumor polysaccharides, blood pressure-reducing angiotensin re-uptake inhibitors and perhaps the highest source of germanium in nature. Germanium is an oxygen catalyst and one of the most powerful free-radical scavengers found in nature.

Organic Lemon Essential Oil: This oil is organic is extracted from the peel and is a rich source of calcium, phosphorus, iron, and vitamin C. The therapeutic properties includes detoxifying, antiseptic, antifungal, fever-reducing, infection fighter, reduces nausea and relieves stress.

Cellulase from Organic Papaya: Assists in digestion by soothing and regulating the bowel. It reduces swelling, inflammation, and assists in detoxifying the body.

Bromelain from Organic Pineapple: Contains protein-digesting proteolysis enzymes. The

therapeutic properties helps to reduce swelling, bruising, relieves heartburn, assist in digestion, and fights infection.

Wild Native American Chapara: Is antibiotic, antioxidant, analgesic, expectorant and anti-inflammatory. The health benefits include treating conditions such as cancer, arthritis, skin disorders and colds. It also assists to improve liver function and is cleansing to the urinary tract.

These high quality ingredients contain a spectrum of vitamin and minerals that assist the body in maintaining optimal health. Getting the proper mineral supplementation is vital for living a long, healthy and active life.

THE IMPORTANCE OF IONIC MINERALS:

I want to go into a little more detail about the importance of minerals. Our bodies are made of the same basic chemical elements (minerals) of which the earth is made.

Minerals are essential and without them, we would just dissolve into little puddles on the floor. Specific minerals facilitate specific functions in the organs and tissues where they are dominantly stored. Each mineral is a conductor or transmitter operating on a specific vibratory frequency. Rarely does an element function alone. Each element achieves its power through bio-chemical combination and relationship with other elements; in other words, minerals all work synergistically with each other.

Minerals have two main functions:
- As an actual constituent of the body in both hard and soft tissue.
- As buffers and catalysts necessary to perform all body functions.

We should understand the importance of minerals. Every living cell on the planet, plant or animal, depend on minerals for their proper structure and function. Vitamins often outshine minerals, but minerals truly are the life-sustaining elements. We could not live without minerals and trace minerals. Here are some important roles minerals play in the body:

- Needed for energy production, cellular maintenance and function.
- Necessary for bone formation and tooth development.
- Ideal for muscle function.
- Vital for enzyme systems, acting as inorganic cofactors which regulate cellular metabolism.
- Required for nerve transmission throughout the body.
- Crucial for hemoglobin production, protein synthesis and the production of hormones.

The importance of minerals required for perfect health has been overlooked. Although your body can manufacture some vitamins, it cannot make minerals. They come solely from our diet and cannot be obtained any other way. Thus a deficiency of minerals is more common than a deficiency of vitamins.

Deficiency symptoms occur when minerals are lacking, which are then resolved when proper balance is achieved. Minerals or elements come from the earth and eventually return to the earth. They can most simply be defined as chemical molecules that cannot be reduced to simpler substances. These main elements essential to health each makes up more than .01 percent of the total body weight. They are calcium, phosphorus, chlorine, potassium, sulfur, sodium, magnesium and silicon. The trace minerals each constitute less than .01 percent of the total body weight and are also essential for health. They are the minerals of iron, copper, zinc, iodine, cobalt, bromide, boron, manganese, selenium, fluorine, molybdenum, vanadium, arsenic and chromium. Other elements contained in the body include some of the toxic metals like lead, aluminum, cadmium, and mercury.

We have heard over the past few years that aluminum is toxic to the human body, that it causes Alzheimer's and a variety of other ailments. Aluminum is actually one of the most abundant elements on the earth. It makes up one seventh of the earth's crust and is always combined with some other element. It is a major component of all life, including our food chain. Beans alone have tested an incredibly high 1,640 ppm. It is in everything we eat but in its natural form. Only when used in excess amounts in this form is it known to be toxic and not for human consumption; the same goes for all trace elements including arsenic, lead, iron and mercury. All are natural minerals that are necessary for human nutrition but can be toxic in excess amounts.

Dr. Linus Pauling came to the conclusion, "You can trace every sickness, every disease and every ailment ultimately to a mineral deficiency." It is believed that most all people are mineral deficient because of modern eating habits. Sadly most of the supplements and processed foods on the market today have been fortified with minerals in the improper form and size for our cells to be able to absorb and use. These supplements and foods are actually harmful for our bodies. It is important to use minerals in the proper ionic particle size. The incorrect size can cause serious problems and health issues. The plants will absorb the small ionic mineral and element. They know it will permeate at the cellular level and "feed" them. When we eat the plant those nutrients enter our body and work in much the same way.

The blood can eventually absorb the larger mineral particles, but because they are too large to be absorbed by the individual cells, they stay in the bloodstream and are eventually deposited in various locations resulting in "heavy metal" build-up. Another problem is the iron particles in breakfast cereals labeled "fortified" being too large for the body to use and can build up and become toxic. Some researchers believe the most efficient way to relieve the body of harmful, over-sized accumulated minerals is to provide the same minerals in a useable form. It is interesting how the body will hold onto the unusable mineral until it receives the mineral in its proper form. This is why you may have a hair analysis done to test your "mineral levels" and be told you have a toxic accumulation of a certain mineral only to literally drop dead a few days later because of a critical shortage of the very same element. This happens because the mineral has not been taken in its proper form. The test simply does not differentiate between mineral levels in a useable form and the larger form that is unusable by the body.

An effective way to cleanse the body of harmful, accumulated minerals is to provide the same mineral in a useable form. This will flush the unusable mineral out. All trace metals introduced to the body in micron or larger sizes cause heavy-metal buildup conditions. Many people go through "chelation therapy" to flush their body of such "heavy metal" accumulations with no successful results, while all they really need to do is provide the body the mineral it was holding on to in a usable form. Another way to rid you body of the "heavy-metals" is by sprouting seeds soaked in water with 1/8 teaspoon of MSM added. The extra natural sulfur has been known to assist in pulling out the "heavy-metals".

Any element found to occur naturally in the soil or plants is organic. It is when man refines out these minerals to use in food products that it changes from an organic or natural form to a synthetic one. When another element is placed with the mineral it becomes a compound such as calcium carbonate, chromium picolinate or magnesium citrate and it is no longer the pure mineral we think we are getting.

Metal poisoning (improper size or too much) primarily affects the metabolic enzymes, brain and nervous system but can affect many other bodily functions as well. In addition to the toxic metals,

some essential elements, such as copper, iodine, selenium, chromium, iron and calcium are more likely than other minerals to cause health problems when high levels are present in the body. The cause is either from excessive intake or reduced ability to eliminate the mineral. All elements are needed and even required to sustain human life but all in trace amounts.

The truth is that the incorrect minerals we consume or the correct minerals we fail to consume have a direct link to everything from acne to the length and quality of our lives. The most important asset we have is our health and it is our responsibility to take care of it. There are many mineral supplements manufactured that are basically harmful. We would benefit by returning to a simpler, more natural way of life. Eat plenty of fresh vegetable, fruits, nuts, seeds, sprouts, berries and herbs. When available, choose organically grown chicken, beef and fresh fish. Finally, get plenty of fresh air, sunshine, exercise and adequate rest.

The following list of minerals is to help you realize how important obtaining them is for your overall health:

BORON: assists estrogen's role in building bones by helping convert Vitamin D into an active form necessary for the absorption of calcium. It is essential to bone metabolism and calcification of bones, and helps prevent osteoporosis, arthritis and tooth decay. It is necessary for cartilage formation and repair. Memory and brain function can be improved with boron. Symptoms of boron deficiency: arthritis, brittle bones, muscle pain, carpal tunnel syndrome, degenerative joint disease, hormonal imbalance, loss of libido, memory loss, receding gums, osteoporosis and weak cartilage. **Natural sources:** whole grains, nuts, seeds, apples, pears, grapes, and leafy greens.

CALCIUM: is needed in every organ of the body and promotes healing. It is valuable for tone, power, strength, longevity, vitality and endurance, healing of wounds, counter-acting acids and helping regulate metabolism. It is one of the first elements to go out of balance when the diet is inadequate. A calcium deficiency is indicated by white spots on the fingernails, is necessary to regain the proper pH balance and leads to a host of diseases and degenerative conditions. When calcium is missing stuttering, stammering, an inferiority complex, soft bones, sores and sore tissues are some of the symptoms.

Other symptoms are: acne, arthritis, acidosis, A.D.D., asthma, Bell's palsy, cramps, colds, chronic fatigue syndrome, cancer, cavities, carpal tunnel syndrome, cataracts, enlarged heart, fibromyalgia, gallstones, and high cholesterol. **Natural sources:** Chinese cabbage, egg yolks, salmon, sardines, white beans, broccoli, almonds, sesame seeds, molasses, maple syrup, tofu, brussel sprouts, collard greens, dairy products, figs, prunes, dates, onions, vegetable greens, kidney and soy beans, lentils, and shellfish.

NOTE: refined sugar and foods high in oxalic acid (spinach, beet leaves, chard, chocolate, cranberries and rhubarb) and phytic acid (germ, bran and legumes) leach calcium from the body and should be used sparingly.

CHROMIUM: a deficiency in chromium is a major factor in the development of heart disease. It helps the body regulate metabolism, regulates insulin, blood sugar levels, assists the liver in synthesis of fatty acids (burns fat) and enhances insulin performance. Some symptoms of a chromium deficiency: anxiety, A.D.D., aortic cholesterol plaque, arteriosclerosis, bi-polar disease, coronary blood vessel disease, depression, diabetes, high blood cholesterol, hyper-insulin, hypoglycemia, hyperactivity, impaired growth, infertility (decreased sperm count), obesity, pre-diabetes, and peripheral neuropathy. Sugar causes the body to deplete chromium more rapidly. **Natural sources:** cloves,

black strap molasses, eggs, dried beans, dulse, potatoes with skins, fresh fruits and vegetables, brown rice, whole grains, meat, and brewer's yeast.

COBALT: is essential to the body in small amounts. It helps repair the myelin sheath, increases the effectiveness of glucose transport from the blood into body cells, help the assimilation of iron and building red blood cells. It increases the body's ability to absorb Vitamin B-12. Symptoms of cobalt deficiency: digestive disorders, fatigue, myelin sheath damage, nerve damage, pernicious anemia, poor circulation, and slow growth rate. **Natural sources:** green leafy vegetables, raw milk, goat milk, meats, apricots, and sea vegetables.

COPPER: the two minerals, iron and copper, work together in the formation of hemoglobin and red blood cells. Anemia can be a copper deficiency symptom. Various enzyme reactions require copper it helps rid the body of parasites, is beneficial for graying and thinning hair. Copper influences protein metabolism, general healing, improves vitamin C oxidation, and is important in the formation of RNA. Low or high copper levels can be found in those with mental and emotional problems.

Symptoms of a copper deficiency: allergies, anemia, aneurysm, arthritis, dry brittle hair, edema, Gulf War syndrome, hernias, high blood cholesterol, hypo and hyper thyroid, hair loss/baldness, heart disease, liver cirrhosis, osteoporosis, oppressed breathing, parasites, Parkinson's disease, reduced glucose tolerance, ruptured disc, skin eruptions or sores, white or gray hair, varicose veins and wrinkled skin. **Natural sources:** liver, whole grain cereals, almonds, green leafy vegetables (turnip, mustard, spinach, kale), black strap molasses, sesame seeds, summer squash, asparagus, eggplant, cashews, peppermint, sunflower seeds, ginger, green beans, potatoes, and seafood.

GERMANIUM: is necessary for optimum health. Low energy and cancer are indication of a deficiency. It raises the activity level of various organs by enabling them to attract more oxygen. It has tremendous anti-fungal and anti-viral responses in the body, creates support for the immune system, and helps correct distortions in the electrical fields of the body. Helps chronic Epstein Barr virus syndrome, leukemia, softening of brain tissue, rids the body of toxins and poisons, reduces high blood pressure, high cholesterol levels and is useful in the treatment of HIV/aids. **Natural sources:** garlic, ginseng, dairy products, onions, seeds, bran, vegetables, whole wheat flour, aloe vera, comfrey, all chlorophyll rich foods, shiitake mushrooms and the Native American herb Tsi-Ahga.

IODINE: is one of the most vital of the biochemical elements and is called the "metabolizer" and mainly affects the thyroid. Iodine restores heat and assists calcium in the repair and building of tissue in the body. Hormones produced by the thyroid regulate and control the metabolism of the body. They also control digestion, heart rate, body temperature and body weight, nervous and reproductive systems. Iodine protects the brain by destroying harmful toxins and helps neutralize toxins in the rest of the body. Iodine helps the assimilation of calcium and silicon. Dry or scaly skin is an indication of an iodine deficiency. Symptoms of an iodine deficiency: acne, cretinism, depression, frustration, goiter, hormonal imbalance, hyper and hypo-thyroid, lethargy, scaly or dry skin, miscarriages, sterility or infertility. **Natural sources:** seafood, yogurt, cow's milk, kelp, eggs, mozzarella cheese, papaya, strawberries, mango, pineapple, and dulse.

IRON: attracts oxygen and builds blood. Along with manganese and copper it is necessary for healthy blood chemistry. It is essential for recovery from illness, assists the body in riding itself of carbon dioxide and keeps the liver tissue soft. Iron combines with other nutrients to produce vital blood proteins and is involved in food metabolism, digestion, elimination, circulation and helps maintain sufficiently high blood pressure. Vitamin C improves iron absorption. Symptoms of an iron deficiency: anemia, anorexia, brittle nails, constipation, dizziness, depression, dysphasia, fatigue/lack of stamina, fragile bones, growth retardation, hair loss, headaches, ice eating (pica), very pale skin. **Natural sources:** red meat, green leafy vegetables (and weeds) especially spinach, kale and beet tops (however spinach and Swiss chard bind iron), beans, lentils, poultry, chickpeas, black strap molasses, chlorophyll, dried apricots, prunes, raisins, dark berries, millet, wheat, sunflower seeds, pumpkin seeds and almonds. Iron from non-animal sources is more readily absorbed if eaten with vitamin C rich foods or a vitamin C supplement.

MAGNESIUM: is a natural tranquilizer. Three hundred enzymatic reactions are dependent on it. Magnesium works hand in hand with calcium to decrease the aging cycle as well as taking the pain out of PMS. It assists in relaxing nerves, relieving muscle tension, helps digestion and is necessary to keep vertebrae in their proper position. Symptoms of a magnesium deficiency: asthma, anorexia, cramps, convulsions, calcification of organs, calcification of small arteries, depression, ECG changes, growth failure, headaches, Kidney stones, migraines, PMS, Malignant calcification of tissue, muscle tremors and tics, myocardial infarction, vertigo, wrinkles, and neuromuscular problems. **Natural sources:** nuts, whole grains, unpolished rice, wheat germ, chlorophyll, pumpkin seeds, navy beans, black beans, sunflower seeds, sesame seeds, salmon, Swiss chard, spinach, and other green veggies.

MANGANESE: is known as the "brain mineral." It is required to manufacture enzymes necessary for the metabolism of proteins and fats and is important in the utilization of all mental facilities/functions. It supports the immune system, regulates blood sugar levels, involved in the production of cellular energy, reproduction and bone growth. Manganese gives us strong nerves, reduces menstrual cramps, PMS, coordination of thoughts and produces elasticity with quick recuperative ability. Signs of a manganese deficiency are: Carpal Tunnel Syndrome, deafness, if due to damage of the cartilage of the ear, ringing in the ears, depression, gout, infertility, lack of concentration, loss of libido in both sexes, memory loss/mental confusion, nerve problems, miscarriages or still births, multiple sclerosis, PMS, poor muscle co-ordination, retarded growth rate, stiff tendons, stuttering, and tremors. **Natural sources:** mustard, kale, collard, chard, spinach, romaine lettuce, brown rice, chickpeas, rye, oats, spelt, the bran/germ of whole grains, black walnuts, other raw nuts/seeds, avocado, maple syrup, pineapple, raspberries, blueberries, and cantaloupe.

MOLYBDENUM: is instrumental in regulating the pH balance in the body. It promotes general well being, aids in carbohydrate metabolism, enhances the body's ability to burn fat, has proven itself useful in MSG (or other chemical) sensitivity, increases libido, beneficial in the treatment of cancer, viruses and parasites. It is a vital part of three important enzyme systems and is necessary for the proper function of certain enzyme-dependent processes, including the metabolism of iron. It also induces sleep.

Deficiency symptoms are: acne, AIDS, allergies, anemia, anthrax, asthma, athlete's foot, Bell's palsy, bladder infection, cancer, Candida, canker sores, cavities, contrail (chemtrail exposure), colds, flu, depression, diabetes, E. coli and eczema. Also Epstein Barr virus, obesity, gout, Gulf War syndrome, hepatitis C, herpes simplex, impotency, insomnia, multiple sclerosis, parasites, liver damage – cirrhosis, lupus, lymes disease, prostate infection and ringworm. **Natural sources:** beans, peas, lentils, eggs, seeds, spinach and other leafy, dark green vegetables, cauliflower, carrots, tomatoes, whole grains (oats, wheat germ and buckwheat), potatoes, Brewer's yeast, yogurt, milk, liver, organ meats, chestnuts, raw cashews, and almonds.

POTASSIUM: is a primary electrolyte, the great alkalizer and is important in pH and water balance. It is vital to the elimination of wastes in the body and

is a natural diuretic that helps your body excrete water and inorganic sodium thus possibly lowering blood pressure. It is critical to cardiovascular and nerve function, regulating the transfer of nutrients into cells and facilitating muscle energy. When potassium levels fall, mental illness and alcoholism may develop as the nerve and mind becomes inflamed and causes the person to only see the negative side of life. When potassium starvation occurs, suicide is often contemplated.

One common sign of potassium deficiency is earaches. Other symptoms are: bad circulation, bluish tint to skin, chronic fatigue syndrome, diabetes, edema, headaches, heart palpitations, hypertension, insomnia, intestinal pain, muscle weakness, oppressive breathing, pain in the eyes, prolapsed uterus, swollen glands, tissue anemia and water retention. **Natural sources:** leafy green vegetables (chard, spinach), citrus, bananas, fruits, black olives, yams, potato peelings, beets, beans, kelp, seafood, crimini mushrooms and whole grains.

SELENIUM: in research has been found to improve the immune system by over 80%. It promotes normal body growth, enhances fertility, encourages tissue elasticity and is a potent antioxidant that naturally reduces the retention of toxic metals in the body. Selenium is critical for the proper functioning of the heart muscle and fight cancer. It works with Vitamin E and enzymes for protein metabolism and healthy hormone balance. It enables your thyroid to produce hormones and lowers your risk of joint inflammation. Symptoms of a deficiency are: age/liver spots, AIDS, Alzheimer's, anemia, cancer, cirrhosis of the liver, cystic fibrosis, Fibromyalgia, fatigue, heart disease, heart palpitations, hot flashes, immune deficiencies, infertility, multiple sclerosis, muscular dystrophy, muscular weakness, pancreas problems, sickle cell anemia, Parkinson's disease, premature aging, scoliosis, and SIDS.

Some symptoms of excess Selenium (toxicity): hinders performance of certain enzymes, can cause hair loss, fever, dermatitis, paralysis, muscular problems, heart problems, increased tooth decay, skin inflammation, nausea, fatigue, liver, and kidney problems. **Natural sources:** organ meats (liver, kidney), seafood, whole grains, fresh fruits, vegetables, button and shiitake mushrooms, and Brazil nuts are one of the most concentrated food sources of selenium.

SULFUR: is known as a healing mineral and assists every cell in the elimination of toxins. It softens tissues, relieves stress, inflammation, asthma, arthritis, Candida, increases circulation and energy, mental calmness, the ability to concentrate and reduces muscle aches. Water soluble sulfur relieves allergies to food, controls acidity in stomach and ulcers and coats the intestinal tract so parasites lose their ability to hang on.

Sulfur has been shown to increase the body's ability to produce insulin, is important for carbohydrate metabolism and speeds wound healing and stops urinary tract infections. Sulfur reduces back pain, relieves migraine headaches, promotes muscle healing, scavenges free radicals and beautifies the skin. Symptoms of a sulfur deficiency: arthritis, asthma, acne, back pain, constipation, dry skin, circulatory problems, inflammation, free radical damage, infection, muscle pain, nerve disorders, stress, skin disorders, urinary tract disorders, various muscle and skeletal disorders, and wrinkles. **Natural sources:** kale, cabbage, onions, garlic, horseradish, egg yolks, watercress, Brussels sprouts, cauliflower, turnips, cranberries, dried beans, legumes, wheat germ, dairy products, meats, organ meats, poultry, and fish.

VANADIUM: is known to regulate the circulatory system, reduce cholesterol levels and buildup in the central nervous system, lowers elevated blood sugar and is believed to help reduce the incidence of heart attack. When used in combination with chromium it is found to be very beneficial in dealing with mineral deficiencies found in diabetics and hypoglycemia. Some symptoms of a vanadium deficiency: cardiovascular disease, diabetes, high cholesterol, hyper-insulin, hypoglycemia, infertility, obesity and pancreatic dysfunction. **Natural sources:** oysters, dill, parsley, radishes, kelp, gelatin, vegetable oil (soy, olive, sunflower, safflower), buckwheat, oats, rice, and green beans.

ZINC: deficiency can lead to a wide variety of degenerative diseases and illnesses. It assists in the proper assimilation of vitamins, normal growth and development, maintenance of body tissues, sexual function, immune system, chemical detoxification, synthesis of DNA and helps reduce healing time both before and after surgery.

It is an anti-oxidant and must be in proper balance to assist some 25 enzymes in various functions involving digestion, metabolism and reproduction. There are at least 60 zinc enzymes in the brain and it is probable that this is related to the observed effect of zinc deficiency on mood states. In monkeys and rats zinc deficiency has produce significant behavioral changes, including aggression. In humans, anxiety and mood disturbances, primarily depression, have been observed in those who develop zinc deficiency during intravenous feeding and in those having an inherited zinc deficiency.

Zinc is needed to trigger over 200 enzymes for growth, immunity and sexual development. Lack of zinc in pregnant women can result in numerous birth defects such as Down syndrome, cleft lip, spina-bifida, clubbed limbs and hernias. Zinc is anti-bacterial, anti-viral and is found in all the body fluids, including the moisture in the eyes, nose, lungs, urine and saliva. Since zinc moves through all the fluids in the body, it creates a defense against infection-causing bacteria and viruses trying to enter the body and stops bacterial and viral replication.

Symptoms of a zinc deficiency: angina, Alzheimer's, anemia, anthrax, alcoholism, acne, body order, anorexia, bulimia, birth defects, cavities, Crohn's disease, depression, diabetes, eye disease, free radical damage, herpes, hypertension, hair loss, infertility, infection, libido, loss of smell and taste, miscarriages, obesity, PMS, still births, thyroid disorders, and urinary tract infections. **Natural sources:** oysters, red meat, liver, egg yolks, yogurt, green peas, spinach, whole grains, nuts, sesame and pumpkin seeds, legumes, poultry, seafood, Brewer's yeast, and mushrooms.

I found deficiencies for the minerals of Gold, Tin, Silver, and Platinum but I couldn't find specific foods. I believe if you eat a balanced diet using the whole foods mentioned for the above minerals you will cover these minerals also. I am adding the information on these minerals:

GOLD: It promotes a general feeling of well being and stimulates the body's natural defenses against illness as well as promoting vitality and longevity. It has been found in improve glandular function and helps the body to relax. It has been shown to have anti-inflammatory effects and many people have reported sounder, deeper sleep patterns where true healing and relaxation takes place. Gold has also been known to repair damaged DNA. Some symptoms of a gold deficiency: arthritis, brain dysfunction, cancer, circulatory disorders, depression, digestive disorders, drug/alcohol addition, gland dysfunction, heat flashes, insomnia, joint inflammation, night sweats, chills, obesity and seasonal affective disorder, and neutralizes fluoride poisoning.

PLATINUM: It is used in Germany by doctors in the treatment of cancer with miraculous results and is believed to be effective in killing disease causing bacteria, fungus, viruses, and helps to boost the immune system. It has been reported to be deadly against the yeast and Candida infections. Many athletes are enjoying the energy boost they feel from platinum. Some platinum deficiencies are: cancer, chronic fatigue, gland dysfunction, back pain, headaches, insomnia and mental alertness, nerve

damage neuralgia, PMS, and poor circulation.

TIN: This mineral is concentrated primarily in the adrenal glands but is also found in the liver, brain, spleen, and thyroid. Tin is found in the tissue and has many chemical and physical properties similar to those of carbon, silica, germanium, and lead. Tin has been implicated in hair loss and hearing loss (ringing in the ears).

SILVER: It is natures most powerful natural antibiotic. When silver comes into contact with a disease organism it actually disables the invading organism's internal functions. It works like a secondary immune system. It can also neutralize sodium fluoride poisoning. Silver is emerging as a wonder of modern medicine. An antibiotic kills some half dozen-disease organisms, but silver kills over 650. Some symptoms of a silver deficiency and some diseases where the use of silver may be beneficial: anthrax, athlete's foot, boils, Candida, Cerebro-spinal meningitis, colitis, cystitis, E. coli, dermatitis, diphtheria, dysentery, gonorrhea, impetigo, infection, influenza, intestinal trouble, ringworm, shingles, staphylococci, tuberculosis, warts, and whooping cough.

Having an understanding of the basic mineral needs in your body and how minerals work is the best way to overcome deficiencies. Remember, it is important that nutritional supplementation be considered part of a long-term health program, not a quick fix. After taking minerals, some people may feel a difference within 48 hours; for others, there is a more subtle change that takes longer to recognize. Ultimately, most people feel increased energy, an improved sense of well-being, and get sick less often.

Good health is being balanced on the physical, mental, emotional and spiritual levels of your being. A key to health is found in maintaining a proper nutritional foundation. Excess or deficiency in any of the primary chemical elements needed in human nutrition could account for most disease and mental symptoms. Human body tissue can neither be restored nor rejuvenated without proper nutritional support.

Eating correctly should be our number one priority. With our highly processed fast food society today it is very difficult to follow a healthy diet. It is even more difficult for our body to digest, absorb and metabolize what we are eating into useable elements necessary for proper body function. The problem is compounded by the fact that many fruits and vegetables are picked green before they absorb the proper nutrients. The soil has also been depleted over the years without a proper balance being put back into it. Nutrient depleted soil equals nutrient depleted food.

Our bodies are not designed to ingest and assimilate foods that are deficient in vitamins, minerals, enzymes, fiber and are loaded with additives designed to give them eternal shelf life. Such "food" leads to sickness and disease. Just as every disease takes time to develop so does eliminating it takes time. In the healing process there is usually a healing crisis. Don't be afraid if you feel you are losing ground for a few days. Gradually, we reverse from the chronic stage of disease toward good health. In the same way our bodies are not designed to ingest and assimilate inferior foods, our bodies do not thrive on pharmaceutical drugs created in a laboratory. More often than not, drugs cause side effects that range from uncomfortable to severe to lethal.

WATER:

Water is the most important nutrient for the body to survive. It serves as the body's transport and reactive medium transporting gases from the body since the diffusion of gases always takes place across a surface moistened by water. It has a tremendous heat stabilizing ability allowing the body to absorb considerable amounts of heat resulting in only a small change in body temperature. It also helps lubricate the joints, giving structure, and form

to the body. Water makes up 83% of our blood. It creates vitality, life and youth as it flows through us, but we need pure water and it must be continuously replaced. An important function of water is flushing out toxins, foreign matter, and excess body salts. A glass of water is like an internal shower. Water should be taken 30 minutes before a meal to assist in weight management and ensure water is not taken from other organs to produce the digestive juice of the stomach.

Next to oxygen, water is the substance we need most. As we age, our bodies harden as we lose the ability to store and to use water. Aging is literally a slow process of dehydration. Most people today suffer from chronic dehydration. Our society has lost the ability to recognize thirst from dehydration. When we feel thirsty, we drink a soda usually with a drug like caffeine or saccharine. One of the greatest causes of human illness is water mixed with other substances, especially caffeine which acts as a dehydrating agent. To compensate for coffee, caffeinated beverages, diet soda, beer and other alcoholic drinks, you have to drink twice their volume in water - and that's in addition to your normal requirements.

Our body needs a minimum of 8 glasses of pure water a day. Feeling tired and sluggish in the afternoon may be due to partial dehydration more than being bored or fatigued. One good way to tell how much water you need is to divide your body weight in half. That is the minimum number of ounces you need (150 lbs. = 75 oz. or about 9 cups). It is also important to know that you body needs more water during extreme cold than it does during hot weather. In the beginning you will go to the bathroom often to relieve the excess water, but in about 4 to 6 weeks your holding organs expand to handle the increased supply.

In today's food and beverage society, thirst is not a valid indication of your body needing water. Instead we need to go by our stomach pains, depression, high blood pressure, high cholesterol, liver and kidney damage, exhaustion, as well as dry lips (a very good indicator), mouth and body pains to know if our body is calling for water.

As you dehydrate from lack of water consumption, the body intelligence constricts lung tissue to reduce fluid loss. It does this chemically by increasing production of a substance called histamine. One of the little known functions of histamine is to regulate water conservation. Drug companies have ads to teach us that histamine is bad and their drug called antihistamines is good. Antihistamines from the drug companies open bronchial tubes, making it temporarily easier to breathe, but they are simply suppressing the body's cry for water and hydration. When the stress of low water levels in the tissue gets worse, the lungs muscular performance constricts making it hard to breathe. This is a signal to drink more water. If you want to see waterpower, have the asthmatic swiftly drink three glasses of water. Water is a wonderful bronchial dilatory and an anti-inflammatory.

Water can revive the sick, elderly, arthritic and those with the flu. It can heal shattered nerves and cure lung deficiencies. It is best to drink pure water throughout the day not all at once. Just as water runs over dried and hardened ground, so it is with the dehydrated body. In time ground can be hydrated just as the body. Chest pain and obesity are signals of extreme dehydration. Profuse water intake will help the body function in its natural process of fluid regulation. Water, not food, should be the emphasis. Water helps headaches. When blood vessels get blocked they constrict and hurt. Dehydration is the cause. Even sinus headaches are helped by hydration. If you do get a backache, one of the easiest and most effective solutions is to drink lots and lots of water.

When injured, the cells in your spinal column need extra water to flush out acid particles created by strain. Also, the natural "shock absorbers" in your back can't function without water to make them soft and spongy. Most back pain can be quickly and vastly improved, possibly even eliminated, by drinking extra water. Try this simple "water cure" and you'll be amazed. Our bodies, minds, emotions, and hearts cry for water. Some people believe high blood pressure is water deficiency. Water improves hormonal functions and can help prevent senility. It calms and helps the emotions and shattered nerves. Water increases physical, mental and emotional energy. Dehydration is one of the greatest producers of free radicalism in the body and water is one of the ways to remove them. Water is for energy regeneration and metabolism.

In a recent study of a major city's tap water, it showed the main ingredient was water and the second major ingredient was shredded toilet tissue. Could it be possible that today's tap water was yesterday's toilet water? Maybe drinking tap water is a slow form of suicide. The report also mentioned that over 40,000 carcinogens have been found in tap water along with parasites. It is important to provide your family with good pure water.

GEM THERAPY NECKLACE and LIFE BALANCE MIST:
We have all had times in our life when we needed to be at our best but just knowing that has created even more stress. What if I told you there was a way to slip into a perfect balance that would allow peak performance in every aspect of your life? What would that be worth to you? The Gem Therapy Necklace and Life Balance Mist create an environment in the body where it can be free of energy interrupters thereby assisting the body to focus on self healing. They protect the natural flow of energy/electricity so the body can perform as it was designed to do. It instantly demonstrates its ability to increase your balance, coordination, endurance, energy, flexibility and strength. The amazing thing is not what the necklace and mist can do for us but what our bodies can do for us given the correct environment.

The human body contains seven major energy centers commonly referred to as "Chakras" where there is focused and concentrated energy. Each energy center has a corresponding relationship to some of the various glands/organs of the body. The energy created from our emotions and mental attitude runs through the centers and is distributed to our cells, tissues and organs. Realizing this brings insight into how we ourselves affect our bodies, minds and circumstances for better or worse. It is up to us to make our choices and decisions in a sacred manner from a place of awareness and balance rather than being blindly influenced by forces we do not understand.

All of the functions related to our amazing body are controlled and coordinated by the extensive nervous system network. It is continually sending and receiving electrical impulses to and from the brain in order to coordinate optimal health. When there is interference or stress in any part of the nerve system it may result in health problems in a variety of different areas throughout the body. The Necklace and Mist along with the Ageless Plus helps to prevent that short circuit process and to correct problems that have already taken place.

Our bodies where created with innate intelligence to maintain health in all areas mentally, physically, spiritually and emotionally. It is the interruptions from the 80,000+ man-made chemicals that we breathe, drink, eat and absorb along with E. M. F. from the gadgets we require for keeping up with life such as cell phones, computers and microwaves that are stressing our lives. The emotional stress of day-to-day living short circuits the electricity from its natural flow and create energy interrupters that affect our body's performance.

The Necklace and Mist harnesses and organizes energy by removing the interrupters. A very effective way to open, activate, energize and balance all our energy centers and keep our body and mind in a healthy condition is by using the Necklace, Mist and Defense as a three part Health System. With this System one area of your health is not sacrificed to "improve" another. It organizes and harmonizes energy instead of manipulating it. Each part is designed to work synergistically providing to the body greater benefits when used together. The Mist works from the outside-in, the Defense works from the inside-out, and the Necklace ties them both together. They are a power-house of subtle energy that works to balance the body in a sacred manner. They are not a cure, prevention or treatment for any disease or malady of the body it simply assists the body to restore balance. They works best when the body is hydrated which allows the energy to flow more effectively.

The Life Balancing Mist was formulated with the intent of organizing particle and wave phenomena related to information processing. It comes in a 4 oz spray bottle containing the essential oils of Rose, Neroli, Roman Chamomile, Frankincense, Ylang Ylang, and Rose Geranium. The Mist works from the outside-in by enhancing the frequency of every cell, healing, bringing balance and harmony to the body, mind and spirit. It eliminates blocked personal growth, stimulates and elevates the mind bringing everything into focus at the moment and creates a sense of well being, peace, and love.

The Mist is sprayed over the head in all four of the traditional sacred directions. As the mist settle around you it clears the aura, is neuro-balancing, supports optimum performance, mental clarity, focus, recall and a peaceful state of mind. The aroma from the Mist relieves stress, frustration, anxiety, depression, fear, nervous tension, indecision and extreme moodiness. It is consoling, gives patience, raises self esteem, and balances the equilibrium and heart functions enhancing relationships. The Mist increases the oxygen around the pineal and pituitary glands, heals emotional wounds, is very calming and soothing to the nervous system and has been beneficial for clearing skin problems. The Sacred Essential Oils in the Mist are known as incredible immune builders, infection fighters, stimulates circulation, assist the adrenal glands, and are a tonic for the heart and liver. It is best used at least six times a day and more often when there are stressful situations to be handled.

The Gem Therapy Necklace is designed with balancing and regenerative functions to assists in stopping energy interrupters and re-establishing the flow of harmonious positive Universal Energy. The stones may be worn as a necklace, placed in a pouch or your pocket. Here is a brief explanation of the characteristics and energies of each Sacred Balancing Stone in the necklace:

Smokey Quartz – Medicine Wheel Position: West – Seeks Council. It is one of the most powerful grounding and clearing stones available. It clears the aura and energetic systems bringing healing energies into the body. It is worn for emotional support assisting in removing mental and emotional blockages, helps to dissolve anger and resentment, relieves pain, and disperses negativity from the body. Smokey Quartz has the frequencies needed to detox and protect from harmful electromagnetic radiation. It is an excellent stone to protect from conflicting electromagnetic energies, such as computers, cell phones, microwaves, and in recovering from exposure to low level radiation sources.

Turquoise - Medicine Wheel Position: South – Looks Within, Hoop – Nervous System. It is known as the "Healer's Stone" and has the ability to heal the body on many levels. Perhaps this is why the Tribes of the Southwest use it as a general body tonic. Turquoise combines the Water, Wind, Fire and Earth energies, thereby containing the power and unity of the Storm element. It "controls" the storm that sometimes rages within us and balances all the systems at once. This kind of balance is essential in today's hectic world, where conflicting energetic messages, coming from all directions at

once, seem to be the norm for many people.

Citrine – Medicine Wheel Position: East – Sees Far, Center. It enhances balance and healing at all levels because of its ability to regulate the Endocrine System. It can be very important in balancing stress, as it levels out the adrenals, and reduces the production of fight or flight Hormones.

Carnelian agate - Medicine Wheel Position: Center – Core Motivation. This smaller cut stone may be of many colors from clear to the red and orange. It lends vitality and energy to the physical body and is the "Core or Corner" stone that gives courage. This stone is the source of the "extra energy" which is often needed in healing or when a new direction is desired. It assists one to overcome the fears that can stop their progress and is very supportive when old, bad habits are to be thrown off.

Carnelian lends courage to "take the leap" and dedicate oneself to a new path. It encourages one to stop waiting for one's dreams to appear and instead begin to direct one's own experiences as channels for Divine Will. It is an excellent support for detoxifying from harmful substances and in breaking negative or hurtful physical habits. It is a positive aid to the Immune System, balances creativity and mental processes.

Unakite - Medicine Wheel Position: South – Looks Within, Center. Its energy is said to stimulate the healing of disease brought on by the repression of emotions, such as cancer (anger) and heart disease (fear and resentment). Unakite supports healthy tissues in general and is particularly useful for promoting the physical health of the heart and the lungs. Its green and pink colors reveal its ability to balance the physical and the emotional aspects of the heart. This stone assists one in truly releasing the negative emotions, the habitual thoughts, and inner dialogue that create them.

Yellow Jade – Medicine Wheel Position: East –

Sees Far. It is a symbol of unity and perfect tranquility soothing the nervous system and reducing stress. It is important in unifying the functions of other stones with which it is placed. Yellow Jade is excellent for physical detoxification, assists the body in maintaining a normal alkalinity, and supports the healing of bones. It balances metabolism and appetite supporting natural weight management.

Onyx Flint – Medicine Wheel Position: West – Seeks Council, Center – Core Motivation. Flint is an Earth Element of amazing power and intensity. Though its primary function is that of grounding, it reaches its energetic tendrils far into the higher-vibrational domains, bringing the highest frequencies of the spiritual into manifestation in the physical world. It is known as the DNA Stone because it "remembers" the First Day of Creation and the original sequences in all things. It settles, calms, and dissipates excess emotional energies. When other stones are placed between the Onyx Flint and Smoky Quartz, they become powerful assistants in restoring damaged DNA.

CLEANSING:

The principle of cleansing is to allow our bodies to restore balance when imbalance becomes too great and threatens our life. Cleansing is your body's natural way to get rid of waste or toxins, and it occurs daily in one form or another. Tears, urine, mucus, and sweat are examples of body cleansing that we regard as very normal. The body has other normal ways to eliminate harmful substances these include fevers, colds, and skin eruptions. We have been taught these are bad and need to be suppressed but this is not necessarily the case. You cannot heal without cleansing.

The cleansing process is very simple. It is the natural force that drives impurities from the body. When the liver, kidneys, lungs, skin, and colon become full of impurities, toxins cannot be eliminated and they lodge somewhere in the cells,

tissues, or muscles. The body then organizes a cleanse forcing the toxins out in some disruptive form like a fever, cold, flu, rash, acne, or other illness. If this attempt to cleanse is stopped by a drug such as antibiotics or cold medicines, the toxins are driven deeper into the body. With each cleansing that drugs suppress, the major organs give up a little of their fight until they give up altogether. Disease occurs when the body loses its ability to cleanse itself and gives up the struggle to remain pure.

When you offer your body high quality, healthy food that is easy to digest, it will respond by showing signs of healing--only to you it may look and feel as if you're getting worse. This is just evidence that your body is throwing out those accumulated toxins. Just stick with it. When this healing period ends you will feel stronger and better.

When you are cleansing get plenty of rest as this helps the body to heal. Eat all-alkaline meals preferably warm such as vegetable soup. Avoid overeating because this diverts your energy from cleansing to digestion. If you crave sweets, satisfy that craving with a few drops of Stevia in warm water. When your body starts cleansing symptoms may get worse. You may have skin eruptions, rashes, vaginal itching and discharge, headaches, flu symptoms, and increased fatigue. The time it takes for the body to cleanse is different for everyone. Cleansing depends on how long the toxins have been in your body and how deeply imbedded they are.

One of the main objectives of cleansing is to have a clean colon free of toxins and waste material. Most people have seven to ten pounds of old fecal matter in their colons, even if they have a bowel movement every day. When this accumulation is removed, the body is free to absorb the essential vitamins and minerals and healing begins. Many people believe disease originates in the colon when waste cannot be eliminated properly. The waste accumulates in the colon and backs up into the rest of the digestive tract, the liver and the kidneys. If the walls of the digestive tract are blocked, nutrients never reach their destination and toxins are absorbed into the body. The accumulation of waste on the walls of the colon provides the perfect breeding ground for disease.

Even if you think you are in reasonably good health, your digestive tract and colon undoubtedly have been abused and will profit from cleansing. If you have a health problem, your digestive tract unquestionably is in poor condition. An initial, deliberate cleansing program followed by maintenance of a clean system is essential to healing and restoring your body. If you start eating properly but don't cleanse the colon, you will slow down the healing process.

We recognize the importance of cleaning our homes and taking our car in for regular maintenance, so why not take care of our bodies? When you begin to cleanse the colon the other organs automatically begin to eliminate their waste into the colon. In this manner, the toxins and waste the body has stored, sometimes for years, can exit normally. To have good health, the body must be cleansed of toxins. It is important to cleanse the bowels because from here toxins are released into the blood stream and travel to all parts of the body. A healthy colon slows the aging process. You can tell what the insides of you look like by observing your skin.

Many people believe that parasites exist only in those who are exposed to unsanitary living conditions. This is not so. Parasites can attack anyone who is in a weakened state and are frequently present in people who have nutritional and/or immune deficiencies. Parasites are difficult to diagnose, can make other diseases, and can even exist without causing any symptoms. Many people do have undetected parasites, the oils to use are Ginger, Fennel, Black Cumin, Peppermint, Tummy Rub, or Freedom Plus.

When you first wake up in the morning, begin your day by drinking a glass of warm water with the juice of half a lemon or 5 to 6 drops of lemon liquid copal. This rehydrates your body from its overnight rest and will help eliminate the acid the body has been cleansing out. Your body continues to cleanse at least until mid-morning, so it's important to aid this process by drinking several glasses of water. Try to get in four of your daily eight glasses by midday. Adding lemon to the water gives it an antiseptic quality and helps stimulate the peristaltic action of the bowels. It is essential to drink pure, good quality water because chlorine and fluoride destroy friendly bacteria in the digestive tract.

Two benefits of a healthy colon are energy and vigor. You might also notice an inner calm, improved mental clarity, the ability to sleep well, and sugar cravings seem to diminish because the body will be better able to absorb the sweetness in foods such as onions, carrots, and fruits. Some people suggest the cleansing process should be used two days a year for each year you are old. For example, if you are 50 years old you should cleanse for 100 days during the year. I believe initially this may be true but as you continue to eat cleansing foods, exercise, get adequate rest, drink plenty of water, and enjoy the sunlight these extensive cleanses will not be necessary.

Babies are born with clean digestive tracts. They build a strong immune system with friendly bacteria. When they eat properly they do not store toxins in their colon and eliminate waste quickly. If we could maintain our digestive tract and colon in the condition of a healthy one-year-old, our life expectancy would be much higher than it is now, and we would be disease-free in our old age.

Putrefaction is the process by which foods decay within the colon and generate toxins and a foul odor. Ideally, the colon should be clean enough that foods spend minimum time passing through it and do not putrefy. Foods that putrefy quickly are the same foods that spoil easily if left out on the counter top all day. They are such foods as meat, fish, and dairy products. These are also the foods that form the most mucus which in turn slows transit time. Fruits and vegetables putrefy more slowly, form less mucus, and are the easiest to digest. Sugar, flour, and dairy products are among the most damaging foods to the colon as they are very mucus forming. The mucus slowly accumulates on the walls of the colon. Even if you eat the healthiest, most vitamin-rich foods available, the mucus barrier will prevent those nutrients from being absorbed.

The colon is the waste disposal unit of the body. If the colon becomes clogged, coated with backed-up fecal matter, or mucous lined we immediately become susceptible to disease. A blocked bowel will back-up and pollute the whole body. When the body becomes overloaded with toxic substances, the blood will dump these poisons in the weakest organ or tissue of the body. When the organ is weak and full of toxins, it cannot perform its natural functions nor remove the toxins that have settled in it. The organ then becomes further weakened so that it cannot fight the toxins and degenerates into uselessness or death.

LIVER CLEANSING:
Once the colon is clean and functioning well, you may want to cleanse the liver since it is the key organ for good health. The liver produces over 500 substances which regulate and control virtually every bodily function. There is a strong relationship between friendly bacteria and optimum liver function. Wherever disease exists you will find an unhealthy liver. If the liver is not doing its job, the rest of the body suffers.

The liver is a large filter and a hard-working endocrine gland. It never aches or "cries" when it is in trouble unless the gallbladder is inflamed. It plays an important role in digestion, the formation of blood, and defending our body against infection. When the body absorbs any substance, the liver intercepts it,

neutralizes the substance, transforms it, or rejects it. If the liver does not alter the nutritive substances we eat, they would all be poisonous to us, even the nutrients from healthy foods.

During digestion, the liver secretes bile to help assimilate fats. The bile lubricates the intestinal walls, regulates the level of friendly bacteria, destroys unwanted and dangerous organisms as they invade the body, and stimulates the peristaltic activity that forces fecal material to move through and out the body. The bile and digestive fluids from the pancreas change fats, proteins, and starches into useful substances. The liver governs digestive functions and must be healed before your digestion, immune system, and overall health can reach an ideal level.

One outward sign of the liver being in trouble is on the face between your eyebrows. You may have one or several deep lines and/or a swollen puffiness. A person with a weak, congested liver barely tolerates the cold in winter and may suffer chills usually following a meal. A congested liver can at times become overactive as it works hard to compensate for the congestion. Then it becomes even more exhausted. If you have an overactive liver, you may often feel feverish and find the summer months very uncomfortable.

A weak liver pulls energy away from the spleen, pancreas and stomach. These organs play a key role in digestion. The intestines are almost totally dependent upon the liver and the bile it produces. Some of the symptoms of a weak congested liver include anemia, hemorrhoids, jaundice, diabetes, eating disorders, hepatitis, loss of appetite, cirrhosis, headaches, dizziness, shivering, sinus problems, adenoids, tonsils, the whites of the eyes become yellow, alternating constipation, and diarrhea.

Other signs are malnourishment and obesity or loss of weight and malnourishment, hormonal imbalance, body deficient in minerals, eye problems such as conjunctivitis, moving spots, myopia, cataracts, farsightedness, astigmatism, double vision, loss of elasticity of lens, and atrophy of cells within eye leading to sensitivity to light.

Skin diseases such as eczema, acne, hives, itching, rashes, and dark pigmentation are other signs of a weak, congested liver. Even the brain and central nervous system are affected when the liver is congested. Symptoms may range from depression, daydreaming, or an inability to concentrate and remember things, to even more serious disorders.

Everything we take into our bodies must pass through this large filter. It stores the remains of all the drugs, vaccines, and medicines we have taken plus the chemicals, hormones, and preservatives from our food. The hormones in birth control pills leave a dark patch in the liver which shows up on x-rays. The fats from dairy, animals, and oily or fried foods are also "fixed" in the liver. Flour products, poor quality vitamin and mineral supplements, improper food combining, and over eating weaken the liver.

Lack of sleep and fatigue from pushing yourself when your body needs to rest weakens the liver. As the liver weakens it becomes more and more difficult to sleep. You will know you have a congested liver if you feel tired and sleepy soon after eating, yet you have plenty of energy about 1-2 A.M. You may tend to worry during this time or have negative thoughts. Digestive problems may bother you late at night and you may have to urinate more than during the day. If you are a pregnant or nursing woman and neglect proper eating habits not only will your liver suffer but also your baby will be born with a congested liver. The constipation of a breast fed baby is an extension of the mother's constipation. It's the mother that needs to be treated.

There are several things you can do to help heal the liver:

- Stop overworking your liver by changing the way you eat
- Sipping fresh lemon juice is very antiseptic
- Rest your digestive tract by eating small meals
- Drink plenty of lemon water and sip vegetable broth or fresh vegetable juices
- Eliminate animal foods completely while you are cleansing because the weakened liver cannot handle ammonia, a by-product of protein digestion
- Stay away from cooking oils and butter because they slow down the liver function
- Eat lightly steamed and pureed foods, chlorophyll-rich greens, and as much raw food as you can.
- Your last meal of the day should be a light one; taken early enough that the stomach is completely empty before you go to sleep.
- Grated daikon (radish) is especially helpful because it takes cooking oil and fats from the body.
- Leeks have antiseptic properties and aid the bile in keeping the intestines clean.
- Asparagus and celery are good liver cleansers
- Carrots help build the blood and encourage the secretion of bile
- Rosemary and Thyme are noted for healing liver congestion

Other ways you can help the liver is to continue to clean the colon, exercise (a daily must), and get more rest; however, don't lie down right after eating a meal if you've over eaten. You need to expend energy until you burn off that excess food.

The emotion of anger is connected to the liver. Holding in anger can further damage this organ, so try to express not only current anger, but release old anger that may be stored in the liver. As the liver cleanses, you may find yourself feeling uncontrollably angry and irritated at just about everyone and everything. The essential oils and my

Emotional Workbook and DVD may assist in learning how to release these pent-up emotions.

The liver is paired with the gallbladder in Chinese medicine and cleansing will strengthen both. When healing the liver all other organs will be strengthened too such as the kidneys and bladder which nourish the liver and the stomach and spleen/pancreas which are controlled by the liver. During a liver cleans, the lower back around the kidneys may ache. The Chinese recognize the connection between the liver and the eyes, knees, and skin. As you cleanse you may have eye problems, your knees may ache and pop, or you have the flu and the liver area may be tender to the touch. Remember though, the Liver cleanse is the most important cleanse you can do.

Remember, the colon must be open and working before you start a liver cleanse. It is very important not to be constipated. If necessary, have colonics or enemas to keep the colon open so the liver can dumps its toxins there. When you are cleansing the liver it is more important to give your body time to rest than it is to do strenuous exercise. Cleansing takes strength, so do very mild exercises during this period. Resume your regular exercise program when the cleansing ends. When using essential oils on a regular basis it is important to eat foods that can assist the liver to stay clean.

DEPRESSION:

Depression is paralysis of the mind. The mind sits on the throne of the body. When your mind can't command, your life has no direction and no propulsion. Depression could be a precursor to a stroke because circulation to the brain is reduced. In an area of the body that is malfunctioning, one of the biggest problems is usually a lack of circulation (blood flow in - to give nutrients to the area or blood flow out - to remove waste, lymphatic flow, nerve circulation, etc). To assist in getting your circulation flowing more effectively through the body you may want to practice the handwriting technique called

"Miles of Lace". It is like making a whole string of 8's hooked together. As you make the top circle on the eight say, "energy up" and as you go down say, "energy down". Do a whole page of this lace for several days for better results.

The brain, like any other part of your body, is not going to work if it is not receiving a good supply of blood or if the blood it is receiving isn't of good quality. The same way that you can have a liver that becomes congested with cholesterol or a kidney with kidney stones, you can have a brain clogged with congestion, mucus or puss. When you feel depressed the first thing you need to think about is getting more blood and oxygen to the brain and getting rid of the waste. Massaging the scalp, ears, neck and shoulders with copals for five minutes will promote better circulation. Several essential oils to choose from would be Circle of Life, Sports Pro, Cypress, Peppermint, Rosemary or Lavender. We seem to hold a tremendous amount of stress in these areas. The muscle that extends from the top of the shoulder to the base of the skull is usually very tense. It is hard to get blood circulating through an area when the muscles are as hard as steel bands.

Generally, people don't fall into a deep depression overnight. Deep depression is like most diseases in that it builds over time but is something we tend to ignore. The circulation enhancing nutrients are the B vitamins. The two main ones that are important for blood circulation are niacin and vitamin B12. Many doctors today believe a niacin flush once in a while is a healthy thing to do. B12 is called the energy vitamin. It assists us with the amount of energy that we have - our zest for life.

The problem is that many B vitamins today are being manufactured from substances repulsive to our bodies. Manufactured B12 comes predominantly from activated sewer sludge or from dehydrated cattle livers that are loaded with bacteria. There is not a more toxic area in a cow than its liver because the liver has the job of filtering out the majority of the growth hormones and steroids that have been pumped into the cow. Brown rice and sprouting grains are the best sources of B vitamins. It is best to use food sources for your B vitamins and since Nature's Nutrients is made from the outside polishing of the brown rice it makes it a wonderful source for **all** the B vitamins. Sprouting your grains or soaking and cooking them over low heat will assist in keeping the nutrients in the food.

There are many causes for depression. A classic sign of depression is, when a person doesn't want to get out of bed. They don't want to get out of bed because they don't enjoy life anymore. Remodeling your home or moving into a new office can sometimes trigger depression. In both of these cases, the toxins associated with all the "new" stuff can cause clinical depression. More people go into depression as they embark on retirement than at any other time in their lives.

A lack of female hormones or constipation can cause depression. Hemorrhoids are a classic symptom of constipation which can causes depression. The person exhibiting these signs needs to cleanse the bowels. It seems as though clinical depression is the outcome of one or more systems of the body being out of balance. Cardiac drugs can cause depression. In the library you can use the Physician's Desk Reference and check the drugs you are using. A large number of common drugs list depression as a side effect.

If you want to get well, avoid watching the news. It is the world's greatest nightmares concentrated into a 30 minute program. Many immune studies today show that (a) your immune system is comprised of components that listen and react to your emotional dialogue and (b) a positive emotional dialogue in your mind enhances and stimulates your immunity and a negative dialogue depresses your immunity. Watching the news is not recommended for depressed people. Learn to focus your life on positive things. Count your blessings and pay

attention to the good things going on around you.

Southern California Edison, the electrical company, produced a brochure about electrical pollution. (This is where the Scalar Energy Cards are beneficial.) It says, "There is electromagnetic pollution and there is a low frequency electrical pollution that is both health hazards. These electrical pollutants can cause many health problems including depression." Southern California Edison advised the biggest polluter was hair dryers because they emit one of the highest amounts of wattage of electricity of any appliance. We hold them next to our brain for long periods of time. They suggested that people limit their use.

Southern California Edison also suggests the light emitting dials (such as the digital numbers that we see on everything from video players to alarm clocks) are a major source of electrical pollution. The secondary problem is most of us having a light emitting dial next to our head when we sleep for eight hours. They suggest we move our alarm clocks away from the heads of our beds and put it across the room. The company that sells electricity is not going to tell you not to use electrical appliances -- unless they have come to the conclusion that your lawsuits could cost them more money than selling you electricity.

The other thing they talked about in their article was portable telephones. They are powerful little units with a massive amount of electrical pollution going right through your head when you use them. The best idea would be to limit your usage. Go back to the old cord. The biggest warning I could find was, "Don't touch the antenna to any part of your body when that unit is on." The final of the big offenders was cellular telephones. Even the manufacturers have now included a warning in the sales kit. The warning is mainly about keeping the antenna clear of your body. Disease is a way that your life is interrupted and you are forced onto a different path. Take the attitude of "what can I learn from this experience and what do I need to be doing differently?" See these times of illness as stepping-stones to new levels of health and awareness rather than stumbling blocks in your path.

EXERCISE:

It is essential to strengthen your body systems through exercise in order to restore a healthy balance. Exercise is as important to improving your health as the food you eat. If the body can maintain a robust cellular oxidation, meaning that virtually every cell in your body is functioning well, disease, and bacteria are killed. When cell oxidation is diminished due to stress, pollution, and junk foods, the body is open to degeneration, fatigue, and sickness.

All other things being equal, what role does exercise play in health? This was the question asked of Dr. Paavo Airola. His answer was "A most decisive role! There can be no health without exercise. It may shock many to hear I consider exercise to be even more important in the maintenance of health than nutrition." He continued, "You can eat the best health foods in the world and take all the vitamins you can afford, but if you do not exercise at all, you will not achieve or maintain good health."

From Dr. D'Adamo's blood types theory, Type O's are very physical beings and they must exercise because they won't get well without it. About 70% of the people have Type O blood and only through exercise can Type O's release their stress and tension. Movement stimulates their minds. If a Type O student needs to write an exam, an hour of hard physical exercise beforehand will help him perform better. When a Type O is upset or angry, exercise will help clear the mind. Type O needs stimulating, hard exercise such as running, handball or cross-country skiing.

Type A and A/B require less vigorous, calmer exercise. Whereas a Type O might swim 100 lengths of a pool, a Type A only needs to swim 10.

Other exercises for Type A are yoga, walking and golf. This type of exercise sharpens the Type A's mind, whereas exercising too much or too hard would exhaust the Type A and create mental fogginess. Type B's are in between. They can balance a day of brisk exercise with a day of calming or mild exercise. Type B's have a wide range in their exercise program.

The mini-trampoline is an ideal form of exercise for all blood types because it requires so little energy but quickly rebuilds the immune system and stimulates the T-cells. Jumping just five minutes once or twice a day is sufficient. If you aren't able to jump then just doing a gentle bounce will work. Exercise adds oxygen which helps kill unfriendly bacteria, stimulating you both physically, and mentally.

WALKING FOR HEALTH:

There is no such thing as the perfect exercise, but if there were walking would be it. If you think about it, that's not too surprising. No matter where you stand on the fitness scale from athlete to jelly roll, walking is good for you. Some doctors claim walking reduces neuromuscular tension better than a standard dose of tranquilizers and prescribe it for emotional problems.

Almost everyone can walk. Maybe you won't be able to walk very far or very fast, but some degree of walking is almost always possible. According to a study at the Tel Aviv University Medical School, "It is possible to improve substantially aerobic physical fitness in three weeks by walking daily with a light backpack load." In the study, those people who were in the worst physical shape showed the quickest improvement. The subjects in the Israeli study walked at a speed of about three miles an hour for 30 minutes a day, five times a week. Research also found that those who walked to music walked 30% longer than those who don't. Contrary to popular opinion, proper walking does not come naturally to all people. Some people shuffle along with their chin folded into their chest. Others use a duck like waddle with their feet pointed awkwardly outward. Many of them don't look as if they are enjoying their walk very much. Their bad habits have stifled and limited many of the rewards they could be getting from their walking. One of the most important aspects of good walking is posture. For many people who have been indulging in bad posture for years, trying to achieve good positioning of the trunk and spine is difficult and requires a great deal of practice before it feels as if it comes "naturally."

In Dr. Wikler's book *Walk, Don't Run*, he says, "keeping your head high, with chin parallel to the ground, shoulders squared backward, abdomen sucked in a little, keeping the small of the back straighter, feet pointing straight ahead." Walking correctly puts less strain on your neck and back muscles and increases your sense of what is going on around you plus it improves the image that you present to others.

Another important point to remember when walking is to keep your muscles relaxed and fluid. When you tighten the muscles unnecessarily you will tire easily. Tension in your muscles will also make you more prone to injury since a tightened muscle has much less "give" to it. When stressed during activity, this lack of "give" puts pressure on the connective tissue around the muscle, heightening the chances of a tear.

When it comes to shoes for walking, the worst thing you can do is have them not fit properly. Wearing poor-fitting shoes can do extensive and sometimes irreparable damage to your feet and body. When you buy shoes, make sure your toes have ample room to move. The best way to measure the space in the toe of the shoe is to stand up in the shoes, wiggle your toes and feel where they are with your fingers. Insure ample wiggle room to avoid painfully blisters from forming on your toes. There you have it – turn on the music and enjoy your walk.

HOW MUCH DOES STRESS WEIGH?

A lecturer, explaining stress management to an audience, raised a glass of water and asked, how heavy they thought it was. The answers ranged from 6 ounces to 12 ounces. Then the lecturer answered that the absolute weight of the glass of water didn't matter but what mattered was how long you try to hold it. If you held it for a minute, that's not a problem. If you held it for an hour, your arm would be aching. If you held it for a day, you'll have to call an ambulance. In each case, it's the same weight, but the longer you hold it, the heavier it becomes.

Then the lecturer explained that's the way it is with stress management. If we carry our burdens all the time, sooner or later, as the burden becomes increasingly heavy, we won't be able to carry on. As with the glass of water, you have to put it down for a while and rest before holding it again. When we're refreshed, we can carry on with the burden. A good suggestion is to find a place you can leave your burdens at night after work and don't carry it home. You can pick it up tomorrow. Whatever burdens you're carrying now, let them down for a moment if you can. Relax, and pick them up later after you've rested. Life is short. Take the time to enjoy it! Here is a cute article I received that shows some ways to deal with the burdens of life:

* Accept that some days you're the pigeon and some days you're the statue.
* Always keep your words soft and sweet, just in case you have to eat them.
* Drive carefully. It's not only cars that can be recalled by their maker.
* If you can't be kind, at least have the decency to be vague.
* If you lend someone $20 and never see them again, it was probably worth it.
* It may be that your sole purpose in life is simply to serve as a warning to others.
* Never buy a car you can't push.
* Never put both feet in your mouth at the same time, it leaves you without a leg to stand on.

* Since it's the early worm that gets eaten by the bird, sleep late.
* The second mouse gets the cheese.
* When everything's coming your way, you're in the wrong lane.
* Birthdays are good for you. The more you have, the longer you live.
* You may be only one person in the world, but you may also be the world to one person.
* Some mistakes are too much fun to make only once.
* A truly happy person is one who can enjoy the scenery on a detour.
* We could learn a lot from crayons. Some are sharp, some are pretty and some are dull. Some have weird names, and all are different colors, but they all have to live in the same box.

SLEEP:

The Stanford University study demonstrated that your internal body clock must be in optimal condition in order for you to learn new information and remember it. The internal body clock guides your daily cycle from sleep to wakefulness and back again may be doing much more than just that simple task. Until now, it has never been shown that the circadian system or internal body clock is crucial to learning and memory. The change in learning retention appears to hinge on the amount of a neurochemical called GABA, which the clock uses to control the daily cycle of sleep and wakefulness.

One of the worst things you can do to disrupt your body clock is to engage in regular night shift work. I realize many may not have a choice in selection of their job but it is vital to understand when you regularly shift your sleep patterns because of a job like police, fire or ER work, then you are simply sacrificing your longevity as if you engage in this shifted sleep period for many years you can easily knock ten or more years off your lifespan.
In brief, your internal clock controls your daily cycle of sleep and wakefulness by alternately inhibiting and exciting different parts of your brain through

regulation of the release of certain neuro-transmitters. The part of your brain known as the hippocampus must be excited in order for the things you learn to be organized in such a way that you'll remember them later. If your internal clock isn't functioning properly, it causes the release of too much GABA, the brain inhibiting neuro-transmitter. According to the results of the study, an excess of GABA inhibits the brain in a way that leads to short term memory problems and the inability to retain new information.

Your circadian rhythm has evolved over many years to align your physiology with your environment. Your body clock assumes you sleep at night and stay awake during daylight hours. If you confuse the situation by staying up very late, or depriving yourself of enough hours of sleep, or eating meals at odd hours (times at which your internal clock expects you to be sleeping), you send conflicting signals to your body. In response, your body will produce 'sleep chemicals' during times when you need to be awake and alert, and 'awake chemicals' when you need rest.

Based on the implications of this study, it's easy to see the relationship between a compromised circadian system, unhealthy sleep patterns, and memory problems – especially in an aging population. Regardless of your age, the best way to keep your internal clock functioning properly is to make sure you're getting the necessary amount of high quality sleep, during those hours when your body expects to be sleeping. The right amount for you is based on your individual sleep requirements and not on a one-size-fits-all specific number of hours.

A good night's sleep is an essential requirement for being healthy, regardless of your age. You can do everything else right – eat nutritious meals, exercise, manage stress – but if you aren't getting high-quality sleep, you simply won't be healthy. Your individual internal clock regulates activity throughout your body, from your brain, to your lungs and heart, to your liver, to your skeletal muscles. Your internal clock keeps all your organs and systems running smoothly. A disrupted body clock can wreak havoc on many areas of your health, including your weight.

Lack of sleep affects levels of two hormones linked with appetite and eating behavior. When you are sleep deprived, your body decreases production of leptin, the hormone that tells your brain there is no need for more food and at the same time it increases levels of ghrelin, a hormone that triggers hunger. Overnight shift work disrupts your biological clock. This disruption may influence cancer progression through changes in hormones like melatonin. Your brain makes melatonin during sleep which is known to suppress tumor development. Melatonin is an antioxidant that helps to suppress harmful free radicals in your body and slows the production of estrogen, which can activate cancer. When your internal clock is disrupted, your body may produce less melatonin and therefore may have less ability to fight cancer.

In addition to the problem with memory reported in the Stanford study, lack of sleep can also harm your brain due to elevated levels of corticosterone, the stress hormone associated with road rage. When your body is under stress, it releases hormones that increase your heart rate and blood pressure. Your muscles get tense, your digestive processes stop, and certain brain centers are triggered, which alter your brain chemistry. Left unchecked, this stress response can eventually lead to a variety of health problems including headaches, increased anxiety, indigestion, insomnia, depression, and high blood pressure. This is another great example of the crucial role sleep and your internal clock play in your overall health and the quality of your life.

Biologists have shown that a functioning internal clock is critical to hamsters' ability to remember what they have learned. Without it, in fact, they can't remember anything. Hamsters whose internal clock was disabled consistently failed to remember their environment, unlike hamsters with normally functioning circadian systems.

SKIN CARE PRODUCTS:
Your skin grows from the inside out, so your overall nutritional levels really matter. Caring for your skin is an outside job too and you can enhance your health by what you are applying to your skin. Your skin is the largest organ of your body and can absorb and excrete both nutrients and toxins through its pores. The condition of your skin is a reflection of just how healthy you are on the inside. The health and quality of your skin is strongly linked to the health of your gut. Taking a high quality probiotic ensures optimal digestive health. Because your skin has the ability to absorb whatever you put on it, careful choices are critical. You want to give your skin the same thoughtful care you give your internal organs. Here are some of the most common harmful ingredients:

Mineral Oil, Paraffin, and Petrolatum -- coat the skin like plastic, clogging pores and creating a build-up of toxins, slows cellular development and disrupts hormonal activity. When there is an oil spill in the ocean, don't they rush to clean it up?

Parabens -- have hormone-disrupting qualities -- mimicking estrogen -- and interfere with the body's endocrine system.

Phenol carbolic acid -- cause circulatory collapse, paralysis, convulsions, coma and even death from respiratory failure.

Propylene glycol -- cause dermatitis, kidney or liver abnormalities, and may inhibit skin cell growth or cause skin irritation.

Toluene – Poison! It is known to be harmful if inhaled or absorbed through the skin. Made from petroleum or coal tar, and found in most synthetic fragrances. Chronic exposure linked to anemia, lowered blood cell count, liver or kidney damage, and may affect a developing fetus. BHT contains toluene. Other names may include benzoic and benzyl.

Sodium laurel or lauryl sulfate (SLS), also known as sodium laureth sulfate (SLES) -- breaks down the skin's moisture barrier, allowing other chemicals to easily penetrate. It can also cause hair loss. SLES is sometimes disguised with the labeling "comes from coconut" or "coconut-derived".

Instead of putting these harmful chemicals on your skin a better plan would be to switch to skin care products made of plant names you can pronounce, recognize, and could even eat. Here are some quality skin care products:

COCONUT OIL – is an ideal way to rejuvenate your skin. It keeps your skin's connective tissues strong and supple offering a youthful appearance by removing the outer layer of dead skin cells. It can even penetrate into the deeper layers of your skin repairing age-damage.

JOJOBA OIL – is very similar to the skin's natural sebum which decreases greatly from about the age of twenty. It's silky, odorless, non-allergic liquid mixes completely and rapidly with your natural sebum and follows its pathways deep into your skin assisting in maintaining the skin's moisture and elasticity. Jojoba oil forms a thin non-greasy lipid layer that holds water in your skin. It contains nutrients that get absorbed into the body, such as vitamin E, B-complex, and the minerals silicon, chromium, copper, zinc, and a lot of iodine. It has antioxidant properties which prevent rancidity giving it a very long shelf life. The Native Americans applied ground seeds of jojoba to scratches to speed healing and minimize scarring.

ORGANIC SHEA BUTTER: is made by crushing the nuts from the Shea tree, yielding nut butter known as Shea butter. Shea butter contains vitamins A and E with antimicrobial and anti-inflammatory properties. The natural healing

qualities of Shea butter are due to the high content of non-saponifiable fats that include keratin, allantoin, and stearic and oleic acids.

These fats help to moisturize and retain the elasticity of the skin that can be used for skin conditions, a sunscreen, wrinkles, scars, and burns by promoting cell renewal and increasing circulation. By using the Shea Butter you can add any of your favorite essential oils to make your own skin creams.

RENEW CREAM: contains – Foraha, Rosemary, and Helichrysum italicum in a base of pure organic Shea Butter. The essential oils stimulate cell regeneration by increasing oxygen circulation to broken capillaries. Renew Cream assists in repairing the damaged barrier function of the skin and helps in retaining moisture. When this barrier is left untreated, it causes dehydration and accelerated aging. It assists in improving the overall health of your skin. It is especially beneficial for those living in a dry desert climate. Apply and massage into the face and neck area after washing.

FIRST AID CREAM: contains the same ingredients as the Renew Cream only a larger amount of the Helichrysum italicum making it very beneficial for healing any type of wounds. It stimulates cell regeneration by increasing oxygen circulation to broken capillaries. Since it is a stronger formula it may burn sensitive skin. Apply a small amount to check. I personally love it.

CUCUMBER CREAM: contains Cucumber Seed oil and pure organic Shea Butter. It is effective in treating eczema, dry skin, psoriasis, acne, sunburns, wrinkles, stretch marks, brittle nails, puffiness around the eyes and revitalizes and detoxifies the skin making it supple and sift. It helps with healing of many illnesses including lung, stomach and chest problems, gout, and arthritis.

The detoxifying effects of the Cucumber Cream helps rid the skin of dirt and oil, thereby clearing up blemishes. Simply applying Cucumber Cream on the temples offers amazing results in reducing stress.

AGELESS CREAM: contains Palmarosa, Rosewood, Elemi, Ylang Ylang Extra, Geranium, Patchouli, Rose and Mink oil in a base of pure organic Shea Butter cream. It improves overall skin health assists with dermatitis, acne broken capillaries, rashes and congested, mature, scaly, or flaky skin. Benefits skin regeneration, scarring, and used to prevent and retard wrinkles, enhancing youthful appearance, and assist skin elasticity. It is calming, assists in slowing the aging process, very soothing for skin problems and wound healing, especially after facial surgery. Ageless assists to re-establish the balance of the skin. It is exceptional when used in place of baby oil. Men like it too as an aftershave cream.

BIRCH CREAM: contains sweet, wild, USA hydro-distilled birch bark oil in a base of pure organic Shea Butter. Beneficial for sore muscle and joint discomfort, accumulation of toxins, sprains, arthritis, cellulites, poor circulation, rheumatism, tendonitis, cramps, hypertension, inflammation, eczema, dull or congested skin, dermatitis, psoriasis, gout, ulcers, broken or bruised bones pulled . It helps in reducing pain and stimulating quicker healing. Use for pulled muscles and other painful unbroken skin injuries.

PAIN EASE CREAM: contains Lemongrass, Birch, and Peppermint in a base of pure organic Shea Butter. It was formulated to assist in reducing pain and stimulating quicker healing. It is excellent when used for inflammation, repairing ligaments, headaches, and circulation. Beneficial for arthritis, sprains, bruises, pulled muscles when massaged into the areas where there is soreness, and pain.

SERENITY CREAM: contains Orange, Tangerine, Patchouli, Lime, Ylang Ylang Extra, Lavender, Blue Tansy, German Chamomile, and Citronella in a base of organic Shea Butter. This cream is great to use on small children and older adults. It promotes relaxation allowing the blood to flow to the brain, is grounding, integrates energy, assists in visualizing goals and dreams more vividly and accurately. It reduces depression, eases anxiety, stress, and tension bringing joy to the heart, balances and stabilizes the emotions, gives patience and calms worries. It may assist hyperactive children in creating serenity in their life. It has been beneficial when used with children that have frequent nightmares and has been known to assist with curing the smoking habit. For insomnia apply to the navel, legs, and neck areas.

SPORTS MASSAGE OIL: contains Wintergreen, Peppermint, Eucalyptus, Basil, Lemongrass, Marjoram and Nutmeg in a base of fractionated coconut oil. These oils were selected specifically for their properties that relax, calm and relieve the tension of spastic muscles resulting from sports injury, fatigue or stress. The Sports Massage was formulated to be used by professionals as well as amateur athletes after, as well as before, workouts or competition. It relieves inflammation, stiffness, sprains, muscle aches and pains, spasms, swelling, cramps and repairs connective tissue. It increases circulation, and assists in supplying energy during stress, emotional fatigue, and physical weakness.

It supports the Adrenal Cortex, stimulates the liver, strengthens cell walls, repairs ligaments, and tones the tissue and muscles. It assists with broken bones (speeds healing), bruises, gout, joint discomfort, rheumatism, arthritis, and headaches. It is deeply relaxing, improves concentration and alertness, strengthens will power, gives a feeling of courage and bravery, and encourages fun and a zest for life. When applied before a workout it will decrease your warm-up time. After a workout rub over all stressed muscles. Massage on the back of the neck to relieve stress headaches. If you will place a hot wet towel over the area massaged for 15 minutes it will drive the oils in deeper for greater relief.

DRY SKIN BRUSHING:

Dirt, dust, pollution, and inactivity cause the pores of your skin to become congested. Since the skin is the largest elimination organ of the body, if the pores are clogged the skin will become either too dry or too oily. Dry skin brushing is beneficial to assist the body in opening clogged pores so the toxins can escape.

Perspiring also helps rid the body of toxins. Taking a hot bath with one of the oils such as Fortify, Spice Traders, Rejuvenate, or Breathe EZ will assist in opening the pores. Using a loofah sponge to skin brush allows the toxins to be released. Using two tablespoons of the dry ginger spice in a tub of hot water has also been beneficial and will increase circulation, cause you to perspire, and the pores to open. You need to sit in the hot tub until you have perspired for a while. About half an hour is good. To eliminate toxins faster, sip lemon water while in the tub and take a cool shower after to close the pores. Caution: Some people get dizzy while sitting in a tub of hot water. Place a cold cloth on the forehead and drink cool water.

ASPARTAME – It is a Poison (an article written by Nancy Markle and shared via email). In the keynote address at a World Environmental Conference, the EPA announced there was an epidemic of multiple sclerosis and systemic lupus. They did not understand what toxin was causing it. The author's lecture at the same conference was about Aspartame (marketed as NutraSweet, Equal, Spoonful, etc) and its link to this epidemic.

When the temperature of Aspartame exceeds 86 degrees F, the wood alcohol in it converts to formaldehyde and then to formic acid, the poison found in the sting of fire ants. The methanol toxicity which can occur mimics Multiple Sclerosis. Thus people are being diagnosed with Multiple Sclerosis in error. In cases of a diagnosis of Multiple Sclerosis, when in reality the disease is methanol toxicity, most of the symptoms disappear when aspartame is eliminated from the diet. We have seen cases where vision and even hearing has returned. This also applies to cases of Tinnitus.

Systemic lupus has become almost as rampant as MS, especially among Diet Coke and Diet Pepsi drinkers. Victims usually drink three to four 12-oz. cans per day. Unknowingly continuing the diet drinks aggravates the condition to such a degree that it sometimes becomes life threatening. When people stop the aspartame, they usually become asymptotic even though lupus is not reversible.

During a lecture Nancy said, "If you are using Aspartame and you suffer from Fibromyalgia symptoms: spasms, shooting pains, numbness in your legs, cramps, vertigo, dizziness, headaches, Tinnitus, joint pain, depression, anxiety attacks, slurred speech, blurred vision, or memory loss -- you probably have Aspartame Disease!" People were jumping up during the lecture saying, "I've got this, is it reversible?" It is rampant. Some of the speakers at the conference were suffering from these symptoms. At one lecture the Ambassador of Uganda told us their sugar industry is using aspartame as an additive! He continued by saying one of the industry leader's sons could no longer walk due in part to product usage!

Another speaker was asked, "Why are so many people coming down with MS?" During a visit to a hospice, a nurse said that six of her friends who were heavy Diet Coke addicts had all been diagnosed with MS. This is beyond coincidence.

There were Congressional Hearings about aspartame's dangers when it was first added to 100 different products. There have been two subsequent hearings, but to no avail. Nothing has been done. The drug and chemical lobbies have very deep pockets. Now there are over 5,000 products containing this chemical and the PATENT HAS EXPIRED! At the time of the first hearing, people were going blind. The methanol in aspartame converts to formaldehyde in the retina of the eye. Formaldehyde is grouped in the same class of drugs as cyanide and arsenic--DEADLY POISONS!!! It may take a little longer to quietly kill, but it is killing people and causing all kinds of neurological problems.

Aspartame affects the brain's chemistry. It changes the dopamine level in the brain. The phenylalanine in aspartame breaks down the seizure threshold and depletes serotonin which can cause severe seizures, manic depression, panic attacks, rage and violence. Every time aspartame is stopped, the seizures stop. There are 92 documented symptoms of aspartame from coma to death. The majority of them are neurological because aspartame destroys the nervous system (phenylalanine and aspartic acid are neurotoxic). This drug also can cause birth defects. In his testimony before Congress Dr. Louis Elsas, Pediatrician, Professor of Genetics at Emory University, stated the phenylalanine concentrates in the placenta caused mental retardation of the fetus.

There is absolutely no reason to take this product. It is NOT A DIET PRODUCT. The formaldehyde stores in fat cells, particularly in the hips and thighs. The Congressional record said, "It makes you crave carbohydrates and will make you FAT." One doctor stated when his patients stopped ingesting aspartame they lost an average of 19 pounds each. Aspartame is especially deadly for diabetics. Physicians think their patients have diabetic retinopathy, when in fact it is caused by aspartame. Aspartame prevents control of blood sugar levels causing patients to go into a coma. Unfortunately, many have died. People have told us about relatives who switched from saccharin to an aspartame product and their blood sugar levels could not be controlled; they suffered acute memory loss and eventually coma and death.

Another physician reported aspartame poisoning is escalating Alzheimer's disease. A hospice nurse told us women are being admitted at 30 years of age with the Alzheimer's disease. This is a quote stated at the conference, "We are talking about a plague of neurological diseases caused by this deadly poison." Aspartame is partially the cause of some of the Desert Storm health problems. The burning tongue and other problems discussed in over 60 cases can be directly related to the consumption of an aspartame product. Several thousand pallets of diet drinks were shipped to the Desert Storm troops. (Remember that methanol is liberated from aspartame at 86 degrees F). Diet drinks sat on pallets in the 120-degree F. Arabian sun for weeks at a time. The service men and women drank them all day long. All of their symptoms are identical to aspartame poisoning. **Avoid drinking diet sodas!**

If it says "SUGAR FREE" on the label DO NOT EVEN THINK ABOUT INGESTING IT! Senator Howard Hetzenbaum wrote a bill to warn parents, especially pregnant mothers and children of the dangers of aspartame. The bill would begin independent studies on health problems such as seizures, changes in brain chemistry, neurological changes and behavioral symptoms. Drug and chemical lobbies killed the bill.

This "poison" is now available in 90 PLUS countries worldwide. Fortunately, speakers and ambassadors at the conference from different nations have pledged their help. We ask that you help too! PLEASE, print this article and warn everyone you know! Take anything that contains aspartame back to the store!

I just learned that aspartame has changed its name. For everyone who wants to keep up on how they slip aspartame into our foods, drugs, vaccines (yes, vaccines), OTC meds (especially child products), aspartame has a new name of **AminoSweet.** Since aspartame has gotten such a bad name (as it should), Ajinomoto has renamed this toxic chemical sweetener. Start double checking your labels. A new product Senomyx, that seems to be just as harmful as aspartame, has been developed by drug technologies. It will remain unlabeled or be labeled as an artificial flavor or flavor enhancer. It has been given the label of GRAS (generally recognized as safe), so it won't be detected like Aspartame (AminoSweet). By receiving the GRAS status given to them by their very own trade association, Flavor and Extract Manufacturers Association (FEMA) they are not required to submit to any rigorous FDA testing on this **drug** that "fools" the tongue so that you perceive that you are eating sugar.

Senomyx is made of such small scale materials that it can fit under the 5% organic standards rule. Kraft Foods who owns organic companies saw to it a few years ago that Congress would change a court ruling that supported only natural ingredients in the organic certified processed products. Now because of Kraft lobbyist "synthetic" ingredients are allowed in certified organic processed foods under the 5% rule. Kraft is crafty...I bet they plan on a line of **dietetic organic food and drinks that will not have to be labeled because it is under 5%.**

ANOTHER POISON – Mono-Sodium Glutamate (MSG): The following is from an email sent me. I think we need get the word out "we are being poisoned." The food additive MSG (Mono-Sodium Glutamate) is a slow poison. It hides behind 25 or more names, such as 'Natural Flavoring.' And is even found in your favorite coffee from brand-name coffee shops!

John Erb was a research assistant at the University of Waterloo in Ontario, Canada, and has spent years working for the government. While going through scientific journals for a book he was writing he made an amazing discovery. In hundreds of studies scientists were creating obese mice and rats to use in diet or diabetes test studies. No strain of rat or mice is naturally obese, so scientists have to create them. They make these creatures morbidly obese by injecting them with MSG when they are first born. The MSG triples the amount of insulin the pancreas creates, causing rats (and perhaps humans) to become obese. They even have a name for the fat rodents they create: 'MSG-Treated Rats.'

This shocking news led John to the grocery store to check labels. He discovered MSG was in everything -- the Campbell 's soups, the Hostess Doritos, the Lays flavored potato chips, Top Ramen, Betty Crocker Hamburger Helper, Heinz canned gravy, Swanson frozen prepared meals, and Kraft salad dressings, especially the 'healthy low-fat' ones. The items that didn't have MSG marked on the product label had something called 'Hydrolyzed Vegetable Protein,' which is just another name for Monosodium Glutamate. MSG is hidden under many different names in order to fool those who read the ingredient list, so that they don't catch on. (Other names for MSG are 'Accent, 'Aginomoto,' 'Natural Meat Tenderizer,' etc.)

It was found that many restaurant items contain MSG. Many employees, even the managers, swore they didn't use MSG. But when we asked for the ingredient list, which they grudgingly provided, sure enough, MSG and Hydrolyzed Vegetable Protein were everywhere. Burger King, Taco Bell, McDonald's, Wendy's, every restaurant -- even the sit-down eateries like TGIF, Chili's, Applebee's, and Denny's-- use MSG in abundance. Kentucky Fried Chicken seemed to be the WORST offender: MSG was in every chicken dish, salad dressing and gravy. No wonder I loved to eat that coating on the skin -- their secret spice was MSG!

So why is MSG in so many of the foods we eat? According to John Erb, in his book *The Slow Poisoning of America*, he said that MSG is added to food for the addictive effect it has on the human body. Even the propaganda website sponsored by the food manufacturers lobby group supporting MSG explains that the reason they add it to food is to make people eat more. It is shocking to see just how many of the foods we feed our children everyday are filled with this stuff.

A study of the elderly showed that older people eat

139

more of the foods that MSG is added to. The Glutamate Association lobbying group says eating more is a benefit to the elderly, but what does it do to the rest of us? MSG manufacturers themselves admit that it addicts people to their products. Not only is MSG scientifically proven to cause obesity, it is an addictive substance. Since its introduction into the American food supply fifty years ago, MSG has been added in larger and larger doses to the pre-packaged meals, soups, snacks, and fast foods we are tempted to eat everyday.

The FDA has set no limits on how much of it can be added to food. They claim it's safe to eat in any amount. But how can they claim it is safe when there are hundreds of scientific studies showing it is unsafe and even deadly. Both the medical research community and manufacturers have known about the side effects of MSG for decades. Many studies mentioned in John Erb's book link MSG to diabetes, migraines, headaches, autism, ADHD, and even Alzheimer's.

John Erb took his book and his concerns to one of the highest government health officials in Canada and while sitting in the government office, the official told him, 'Sure, I know how bad MSG is. I wouldn't touch the stuff.' But this top-level government official refuses to tell the public what he knows. The big media doesn't want to tell the public either, fearing issues with their advertisers. It seems that the fallout on the fast food industry may hurt their profit margin.

The food producers and restaurants have been addicting us to their products for years, and now we are paying the price for it. Our children should not be cursed with obesity caused by an addictive food additive. The best way we can help to save ourselves and our children from this drug-induced epidemic is to share this article with others. We need to stop being rats in one giant experiment. Stop approving of foods that makes us into a nation of obese, lethargic, addicted sheep, feeding the food

industry's bottom line while waiting for the heart transplant, the diabetic-induced amputation, blindness, or other obesity-induced, life-threatening disorders. Blowing the whistle on MSG is our responsibility.

HIGH FRUCTOSE CORN SYRUP (HFCS):
Here is just another giant food industry cover up that might make you want to go all raw and natural. They are sneaking into our foods high fructose corn syrup (HFCS) that is acting as a secret addictive culprit to encourage overeating which in turn sells more products. The Department of Agriculture data directly links HFCS to skyrocketing diabetes and obesity. The food industry started using HFCS because it's much cheaper than regular sugar. Only later did they find it makes you hungrier. Biting into a super-sized burger makes you hungrier than before, even though it technically fills your belly.

HFCS is not a natural product either like I was first told. In fact, I use to tell people not to worry about it because it was a natural sweetener. How wrong I was! It's an additive "designer chemical" that's killed more people than heroin. And it is silently being added to hundreds of best-selling foods. Enough is added each year so that the average American is unaware they have swallowed more than 56 pounds. It is a killer in "natural" disguise. It is made from corn starch. The corn starch is put into vats of murky fermenting liquid, fungus, genetically modified enzymes, ion exchange and lots more chemical tweaking takes place in one of 16 huge chemical plants located in the Corn Belt.

A study shows that 9 out of 10 adult men and 7 in 10 women will become overweight before they die. The drug companies are counting on the increase of obesity and diabetes and are already spending millions to build some of the largest factories ever devoted to making a single drug – Insulin. They see the writing on the wall. It is almost the perfect crime. Most people aren't even aware that the murderer exists! Even if you are trim now you are doomed to balloon unless you stop your intake of HFCS. HFCS acts exactly like an "anti-diet pill," raising your levels of the very same make-you-fat hormones that diet pills are engineered to block. It makes your body ravenous.

Unlike table sugar, HFCS doesn't trigger the release of leptin, the substance that makes you feel full and stop eating. Worse still, it doesn't suppress the release of ghrelin, the substance that makes you hungry. In other words, you feel hungry and never feel full no matter how much you eat. That's why you can't help wanting to consume more food. Learn to listen to your body. If you feel hungry after eating an adequate meal, know you have probably eaten HFCS just learn to read labels.

Between the years of 1970 to 1990 the amount used by manufactures increased by 1000%. There has been no other food or food group whose intake has increased so fast. But there's a big-time cover-up! Since 2006 there has been a big PR campaign just to deny the facts mentioned above. The HFCS is helping the manufactures sell billions of dollars worth of food you'd never crave otherwise.

The HFCS isn't just in soda and gummy bears it is even plentiful in foods hyped as "natural" and "healthy" including many breads, whole grain cereals, fruit juices, iced tea, yogurt, energy bars, spaghetti sauce, salad dressings, and endless varieties of snacks. It would be far better to put a little refined sugar on your oatmeal than eat a packaged "natural grain cereal" loaded with HFCS.

According to Dr. David G. Williams, the great news is that avoiding this chemical could be the only "diet pill" you ever need. If you want to cure the cravings that cause obesity and diabetes, just say no to HFCS. You may be amazed how quickly your weight and blood sugar problems improve.

ENERGY CENTERS:
The human body contains hundreds of locations where there is focused and concentrated energy. There are, however, seven major energy centers commonly referred to as "Chakras" which means "wheels." The chakras are similar to wheels in that they are spinning vortexes of energy. They are centers of force located within our body through which we receive, transmit and process life energies. Each chakra in the body is recognized as a focal point of life force relating to physical, emotional, mental, and spiritual energies. Each energy center has a corresponding relationship to some of the various glands/organs of the body.

It is important to understand the energy centers are "doorways" for our consciousness. They are doorways through which emotional, mental and spiritual force flow into physical expression. The energy created from our emotions and mental attitude runs through the centers and is distributed to our cells, tissues, and organs. Realizing this brings tremendous insight into how we ourselves affect our bodies, minds, and circumstances for better or worse. Understanding this will enable us to make our choices and decisions from a place of awareness and balance rather than being blindly influenced by forces we do not understand.

Here is a brief explanation of the locations of the seven major energy centers or chakras, their colors, and the essential oils that may be beneficial to use on each location:

1. Root or Base Center is located at the base of the spine (coccyx); Cedarwood, Myrrh, Patchouli, Cinnamon Blend, Hormone Balance; the color is Red.

2. Naval Energy Center is located in the lower abdomen to navel area; Jasmine, DNA Repair, Creamsicle, Sandalwood, Rose, Forgiveness; the color is Orange.

3. Solar Plexus Energy Center is located above the navel and below the chest; Lemon, Cinnamon Blend, Grapefruit, Bergamot; the color is Yellow.

4. Heart Energy Center is located in the center of the chest; Rose, Melissa, Ylang Ylang, Love, Forgiveness, Grateful; the color is Green.

5. Throat Energy Center is located in the throat area; Confidence, German Chamomile, Eucalyptus, Myrrh; the color is Sky blue.

6. Brow Energy Center is located in the center of the forehead; In The Moment, Rose Geranium, Peppermint, Focus, Brain Power; the color is Indigo (dark blue).

7. Crown Energy Center is located at the top of the head; Frankincense, Rosewood, Lavender, Juniper Berry, Rosemary; the color is Violet.

There are also powerful energy centers in the palm of each hand and on the sole of each foot. It is good to eat fresh fruits and vegetables rich with the corresponding colors of the energy centers and live your life in alignment with honesty and complete integrity.

The most powerful way to open, activate, energize, and balance all our energy centers and keep our bodies and minds in a healthy condition is to love ourselves and others unconditionally. This may not appear to be a very scientific technique, but it is. Love is the greatest healer. Love is the vitalizing, nourishing, and sustaining electricity of life. We really have no choice over who is going to love us. We only have a choice of who we are going to love. Loving others is our choice. When we love ourselves and are able to offer this love to others, we keep our body/mind systems charged and vitalized with this "electricity."

To love others and ourselves unconditionally may sound like a difficult thing to achieve, but in reality it can be as simple as believing it is possible! Once we experience unconditional love, we awaken the desire within ourselves to move into this state of being. We can begin to manifest this reality in our

lives immediately! Love is a choice. Love is the source of all healing and it is a commandment of God. He said, "The second great commandment is to Love one Another"!

Consciously expand your expression of gratitude, unconditional love, compassion, forgiveness and creativity. Selfless service will aid the opening of the energy centers in a natural and non-forceful manner. Your reality is what you choose it to be!

NOTES FROM WORKSHOPS

When an essential oil is referred to as "**Neat**," it means the oil has not been diluted with anything. It should be a single species and as pure as it was when it was distilled without chemicals.

A **"Synergy"** is when the combination is more than the sum of the parts. When you mix together two or more "neat" oils, you are creating a chemical compound different from any of the component parts. Thus, synergies are very particular and powerful. An increased potency can be achieved by synergistic blends without increasing the amounts of oils used. For example, the anti-inflammatory action of Chamomile is greatly increased by adding Lavender. The interaction of particular oils upon each other increases the whole vibrancy of the synergy which could not be achieved by using a single component on its own.

Blend - A blend is like a synergy except the "neat" oils have been combined with carrier oil for two reasons. One is to keep the "hot oils" from burning when applied and two it keeps the cost more affordable on the very expensive oils such as Rose and Neroli.

The fastest way to get the benefits of essential oils is through smell. The only thing that affects the amygdala where the memory of events is stored is through the sense of smell.

Focus essential oil may raise the brain frequency. Use it for pushing, opening, and awakening the brain. Adding a few drops of Lemongrass is good for the mind.

In Japan an experiment was conducted diffusing various essential oils in the office. It was noted that when they diffused lemon there were 54 percent fewer errors, with jasmine there were 33 percent fewer errors and with lavender there were 20 percent fewer errors among their staff members.

When an essential oil was diffused while studying and the same oil was diffused during a test, the test scores increased by as much as 50 percent. The smell of the oil may bring back the memory of what was studied.

A mixture of Lavender and Grapefruit diffused in the office has been known to keep the staff on their toes, even-tempered and relaxed.

There are different grades of essential oils. One main difference between the grades is the time and temperature during distilling. When Lavender reaches 280 degrees the oil will fracture. The fragrance will still be there but the essential oil is ineffective or even toxic.

A mixture of Lavender, Bergamot, and Geranium will alleviate depression and anxiety. One drop of Neroli under the tongue has been effective for depression.

Use Confidence first on the feet before using other essential oil since it assists all other oils used in being more effectiveness. Confidence keeps electrical fields balanced and gives courage to stand up for your values, especially when you are afraid.

Juniper Berry, Lime, Lemon, and Rosemary are good for energy, control, and focus. People who are under extreme stress tend to be much more susceptible to illness. Where there is no caring there is no healing. Could this be because the body pH is out of balance?

If you are in a state of fear you will never have good health. Fear and emotions can drain energy. With fear your blood vessels tighten up and oxygen and nutrients can not get into the cells. To assist others you must overcome fear.

If you want to change the physical body you need to change the electrical fields first. Essential oils and minerals will help.

For a wonderful bath salt use ten drops of Love in some Epsom salts.

Scientists know that black cumin stimulates bone marrow, immune cells, raises the interferon production, protects the body against viruses, destroys tumor cells, and inhibits infection. It encourages the gallbladder to flush out toxic deposits and to maintain proper bile flow. According to scientists at the Cancer Immuno-Biology Laboratory of Hilton Head Island, South Carolina, Black Cumin has proven to be more effective than chemotherapy and radiation treatments — without their serious side effects.

Thought forms build beliefs. Become aware of your thoughts because what goes out on that frequency will bring back to you ten fold. It is not good to send out bad thoughts because you can't stand ten fold coming back. Life is our examination.

You cannot have hot thoughts (prosperity) and cold thoughts (lack of money) at the same time. Build the replacement to get rid of the negative thoughts. Take away the energy from the wrong thought by not concentrating on it. Concentrate on what you really do want. It is all right to define the problem and then determine if you are feeding it, then build a solution and empower that solution.

When someone around you is negative, reflect it back to them by pretending to put a mirror around yourself. That way you are not giving them more negatives, but just sending back what they gave out. Or you may choose to send back love to change them. Everything that happens to you reveals your thoughts. You attract what you think about. It's important to keep your thoughts on what you want to be in your life.

For bone spurs one person used Breathe EZ on location and had good results.

Drinking water, eliminating soda or sweetened juice has been helpful for back problems.

If you use Vitality and your appetite goes up, it may be because you are not assimilating what you are eating. Look at getting more enzymes in you diet. In 1992 it was reported that over 5,000,000 men and women weighed over 500 pounds in the USA. In 1982 researchers at John Hopkins University calculated that Americans had bought into 29,068 theories, treatments and schemes to lose weight.

Premature aging is caused by a lack of oxygen. Oxidants are poisons and the more you are exposed to them the older you will look. As you oxidize you lose enzymes. Using antioxidants and enzymes are important to stay young looking. Selenium is a mineral antioxidant that should be included in your daily supplementation because it enhances many of the other antioxidants.

Once you get around 40 years old you need more exercise to slow down the aging process.

After applying a single oil it is good to use either carrier oil or a blend that contains carrier oil last so it will seal in the oils so they won't evaporate as quickly.

Using extra pH Rescue for two weeks before doing emotional work will provide more electrolytes to assist the emotional work. Rubbing your feet with Dreamtime will help continue the emotional work while you are asleep.

Break Thru was formulated to help release anger from the liver where these emotions are stored. When working with the emotions, put Confidence on the feet first for balance, Serenity behind the ears, Love over the navel and on the liver and then Break Thru on the feet. You may also want to smell the Break Thru and apply it over the liver. When you are using essential oils for emotional release, please use only a few at a time because you may not want to release stored emotions too quickly.

The Breathe EZ and Resp EZ are very powerful for the lungs. In a small room diffuse either one at high speed. Put a compress of Breathe EZ or Resp EZ on the chest and back. Don't worry if the sick person starts throwing up, it is only a quicker way the body has of clearing out the lungs.

Thyme is a good free radical scavenger.

Confidence and True Blue applied on the back have worked wonders for all types of back problems. If it doesn't reduce the pain significantly, it could be caused by emotions.

Another thing that will clear up a bruise is to rub the inside of a banana peel over the area.

We build a life by what we give. To perform beyond your limits you must first think beyond them.

It is good to drink celery juice while detoxifying heavy metals because it soothes the mucus membranes.

When you go to the location were there is discomfort, run your hand over the area and feel the energy exchange. When there is stress in the muscle, it is hot. Pain in the left shoulder means gall bladder and the right shoulder is the liver.

Burning pain is always nerves. Wherever there is a block in your energy field there will be pain.

If you get a headache when using the copals you have stirred up toxins that are now ready to be released from the body. Drink a lot of water.

Kind words can be short and easy to speak, but their echoes are truly endless. – Mother Teresa

Here are some of the ways to use the liquid copals:
- Birch is for bones. Apply the copal by massaging the "spine" area on the feet.
- Marjoram is for muscles.
- Basil is for inflammation.
- Cypress is for circulation.
- Helichrysum italicum is for nerves.

- Peppermint is for inflammation and to waken the nerves.
- Juniper Berry and Geranium are for reconnecting nerves.
- Rose is the number one copal for emotional healing. Apply over the heart and inhale.

Putting Migraine Relief on the temples and the back of the neck is beneficial in relieving a headache. True Blue is also good for any type of discomfort.

For people who are negative towards the copals, start out easy. Essential oil may make a negative person who does not want to change more negative.

Tangerine has been beneficial for shrinking tumors by rubbing it over the area. It contains certain chemical constituents that have been known to shrink cancer.

Carrot seed copal stimulates the regeneration of liver cells.

Blend five drops of Sport Pro with three drops of Birch in carrier oil and apply on sinus areas. Next put your hands over the nose and breathe deeply to clear the head and open the sinuses.

Hair loss is caused by an imbalance in the hair. Mix together two drops each of the essential oil of Lavender, Sage, Ylang Ylang, and Rosemary then massage into the scalp. Leave it on all night and wash out in the morning. Daily application is best. Some like to use Holy Basil and Hair Support together.

Essential oils that have been found to help when you are ending a relationship are Cypress, Spruce, Juniper Berry, Orange, Tarragon, Guardian, Love, Grateful, Confidence, and Mountain Retreat.

For those living in the South or have a fire ant problem, the Urban Harvest of Houston has come up with an environmentally friendly solution. Here is their suggestion: one gallon of water, one tablespoon of molasses, one squeeze of liquid soap, and 6 ounces of citrus oil (they suggest orange oil).

Plant enzymes taken on an empty stomach enter the bloodstream where they assist the immune system by digesting, disposing of toxins or any other substance that does not belong in the blood, and "eating" the protein coating on certain viruses enabling immune system workers to then destroy them. Thus, taking plant enzymes in this way can help reverse inflammation. It is estimated that enzymes are facilitating 36 million biochemical reactions in the human body every minute. Some of the best food sources of enzymes are avocados, bananas, papaya, mangoes, pineapples, and sprouts. Whenever there is stress there are low enzymes.

Vitamin and mineral deficiencies may result from a refined food diet or the inability to digest whole foods. Combining small amounts of foods high in the desired nutrients with the plant enzymes required to digest them may assist in getting the nutrients from the food. In this way the nutrients have a much better guarantee of reaching the cell and relieving nutritional deficiencies than taking some isolated vitamins or minerals supplement.

There is evidence that if your liver needs cleansing you will hold on to unwanted weight. You may want to try a liver cleanse at least once a year.

Microwave ovens affect your health in two ways. First, by emitting electromagnetic radiation into your immediate environment and secondly, by destroying not only the enzymes in the food but also the nutritional value of the food itself.

Sandalwood has helped fallen arches.

BGH (bovine growth hormone that is genetically engineered) can completely deplete your body of enzymes as your immune system tries to counteract the immune-suppressing impact of the hormone. It is difficult to avoid BGH unless you buy organic dairy

and beef. This would be another reason to supplement with the plant enzymes.

Spikenard has been used successfully to replace valerian.

Minerals assist in relieving depression.

It is important to get your minerals daily. I just read a statement that said, "The organs get the first minerals, then the skin and then the hair."

If you have allergies, fatigue, bloating, gas, constipation, indigestion or any symptom of undigested food then you most likely have an enzyme deficiency. Undigested food becomes a poison in your body.

Fear and emotions can drain energy causing exhaustion. Exhaustion is the manifestation of glands needing to be oxygenated. Work on the big toe with Peppermint, or Focus essential oil and use Spruce on the center of the foot over the adrenal area. If you have more time apply Peppermint and Eucalyptus to these five areas: wrists, ankles, knees, shoulders and elbows. Wrap with moist towels. This takes the "hot" energy from the body when there is exhaustion.

For energy, put a couple drops of Rosemary in your mouth and wash it down with water.

Roman Chamomile is excellent for emotions. The esters in this copal work very deep and high in the mind to unblock emotions.

Research indicates that when the pH level is between 7.0 – 7.5 viruses and harmful bacteria become inactive and at 8.0 – 8.5 they die.

If you have a big belly you probably have parasites. Itching ears, nose and armpits may be parasites. Eating pomegranates, grapefruit and other tart fruits have been known to kill parasites.

In general, oils with sesquiterpenes alcohols tone the muscles, nerves, reduce congestion in the veins as well as in the lymphatic system and have moderate antimicrobial effects. Such oils are German Chamomile, Ginger, Patchouli, Carrot Seed, Sandalwood, Peppermint, Sage, Vetiver, and Spikenard.

If you need to get right into a specific area, use copals that are high in phenols such as Thyme and Oregano. Phenols act like the sharp point of the knife and get to the source. Phenols can be hard on the liver so if you use them often it is important to do a liver cleanse.

Coriander (Celentro) is said to pull out heavy metals. Sandalwood is traditionally used for bladder or urinary tract infections and heartburn.

Dr. Penoel has said, "Cancer is a disease and you need the body pH balanced. It is what you eat, think and feel. Cancer means 'I want to kill myself'. Whenever there is cancer ask them about this. Tea Tree and Lavender make a nice blend to use. The sole of the feet is the safest way to apply oils."

The minerals work together and are best taken in a complete ionic form. Copper helps iron.

Germanium corrects electrical fields. Molybdenum is necessary for the metabolism of iron and raises the body pH. Use boron to help grown new bone under the gums. Vanadium regulates the circulatory system. It is interesting how everything works together in the body.

For breaking up large bruises use - One drop Hyssop, two drops Bay Leaf and three drops Birch.

The prophet Mohammed stated that Black Cumin cures every illness except death. Black Cumin was once highly valued as a healing plant.

A weakened immune system is a modern disease brought on by constant stress, poisons in our environment, severe psychological strains, a lack of sleep or physical activity and an unbalanced diet.

Clear up the pancreas and your eyesight will improve.

The skin is the largest elimination organ of the body. It should be kept "open" by daily skin brushing and a good ginger bath once in a while.

A high protein diet is over stimulating to the body and can cause serious damage. When the diet consists of more protein than is needed, enzymes in the liver and kidneys break down the excess. The major by-product of protein breakdown is urea which is a diuretic. This causes the kidneys to urinate more fluid. Along with water, minerals are lost in the urine. One of the most important losses is calcium.

Experiments have shown that when subjects consumed 75 grams of protein daily, even with an intake as high as 1400 milligrams of calcium, more calcium was lost in the urine than was actually absorbed. This deficiency must be made up by the body's calcium reserve which is taken from the bones. Deficient bones are a stepping stone to osteoporosis. The experiments all showed that when excessive amounts of protein or food in general are eaten, there is a corresponding decrease in enzymes, vitamins, and minerals.

Signs of a mild liver dysfunction include a bloated feeling, foggy brain, and bad breath.

Turpentine is used to adulterate many essential oils.

Not enough attention is placed on taking plant enzyme supplements or eating raw food. When we do not replenish our enzyme level and only take vitamins and minerals, it is self-defeating. The body has to replace enzymes from within, stealing enzymes from all parts of the body which in the end causes exhaustion, premature aging and low energy. When our enzyme level is lowered, our metabolism is lowered and so is our energy level. It is very important to use only plant enzymes.

A few drops of Cloves Bud on an ant bed will kill the ants.

For insect bites use the oils of Lavender or Purify dotted directly on the bite. Avoid rubbing since this will spread the poison from the bite.

Cypress has helped for nosebleeds. By putting a couple of drops of Cypress on a tissue and putting it into the nose, the bleeding was stopped very soon.

Cypress has been used for toenail fungus with good results.

A few drops of Lemon, Eucalyptus, Peppermint, First Aid, or Purify can be added to the dishwater or washing machine to help purify and disinfect.

Pure liquid copals are natural, refreshing and healthy alternatives to synthetic fragrances and deodorants. Good copals to use as a deodorant are Citrus Passion, Cedarwood and Eucalyptus.

Two drops Orange and one drop Peppermint in 24 oz. of water is known to assist an upset stomach.

Five drops of Spruce combined with two drops of Cedarwood and one drop of Peppermint in ¼ ounce of FCO strengthens the functions of the adrenal glands without over stimulating them the way coffee does. This blend applied all over the body, after the morning shower, will act as a substitute for morning coffee.

Some women have told me that putting a drop of Neroli under the tongue has been more beneficial for them than taking Prozac.

Every disease is caused by a mind not at ease.

Unforgiving is the most prolific cause of disease. It will harden arteries or liver and affect eye sight. In its train are endless ills. Use the Love to move

through the emotions of not wanting to forgive.

Sage is used to stimulate bile production.

Melissa seems to be one of the strongest antiviral agents available in the oils.

Tangerine breaks down cellulite fat pockets.

Lemon is perhaps the most effective oil for disinfecting the air using a diffuser.

Lavender normalizes the liver's blood sugar output. One or two drops of Lavender noticeably reduce the appetite when taken 15 minutes before a meal.

Neutralize the odor of stinky feet naturally by using Sage or Tea Tree oil. Sprinkle one of them in your shoes and you'll soon say good-bye to stinky feet.

For a sore throat put one drop of Spice Traders on your finger and apply inside your mouth on the sore area of the throat. It is a little spicy but it does the trick. If you apply it soon enough, only one application is needed.

For dandruff dab some Thyme oil diluted with olive oil (3 drops of thyme per teaspoon of olive oil) on your scalp one hour before washing your hair. After shampooing, it's thyme for an anti-dandruff rinse. To make the rinse, boil a handful of dry thyme leaves in one quart of water, strain, cool, and rinse your hair.

Circle of Life and Neem Plus are beneficial for hemorrhoids. For a few days apply several drops right on location.

Three of my favorite oils for insomnia are Lavender, Valerian, or Serenity. Just apply a few drops to the temples, under the nose and the calves of your legs. Also, to get the stress out take a pen, a piece of lined paper and do a page of "push-pulls." This is just a simple line up and down between the lines on the paper. It looks like a lot of sharp pointed M's hooked together across the page. It really works.

The Mediterranean secret for restoring vitality is 3 or 4 drops of Peppermint oil added to one tablespoon olive oil and massage into your feet.

The first thing in the morning, swish one large teaspoon of cold pressed sesame seed oil around in your mouth for 15 minutes. This assists in pulling the toxins that have accumulated in the mouth, cheeks and face area out into the oil. It has been known to be beneficial for acne, complexion, sore gums and sore throats. After the 15 minutes spit the toxic sesame seed oil into the toilet, flush it away and then brush your teeth and tongue. You will begin to see results within just a few days. Some people with skin problems use this technique three times a day. It is best to do on an empty stomach first thing in the morning.

Many people are deficient in potassium from not eating enough fruits and veggies and consuming a lot of sodium in processed foods. A great source of fiber and potassium is figs.

Fresh parsley is a flavorful way to add significant amounts of trace elements such as copper, magnesium, molybdenum, and zinc to your soups, stews, sauces, vegetables, and salads.

Zinc is the single most nutritional deficiency in North America. Major sources of zinc are whole grain breads and cereals. Refined white flour and sugar have no zinc and deplete the body of B vitamins.

A study in the American Journal of Clinical Nutrition found that people who ate foods rich in Vitamin C had fewer wrinkles and less age related dry skin than those who had a diet low in Vitamin C.

A quick relaxation technique is to breathe in and shrug your shoulders lifting them towards your ears and then as you breathe out, completely relaxing all the muscles from your neck to your shoulders, across your upper chest and upper back and say Ahhhh.

Mismanaged stress can affect your immune system, heart function, and nervous system, reduce mental clarity and memory, increase blood pressure and lead to pre-mature aging. Harvard study showed people who coped poorly with stress became ill more often than those who coped well with stress.

To improve your mood, reduce stress and gain health, smile and laugh often. As you laugh your brain will release endorphins which will make you feel good.

To keep your mind sharp and memory intact as you age, find ways to challenge your mind. Play stimulating games, take up a new hobby, learn something new, or change your daily routine.

Harvard researchers have found that low light levels stimulate the pineal gland to secrete melatonin. Keep the lights low for a few hours before bedtime can help you fall asleep easily.

Licorice root is the dried root of the licorice plant. For the purpose of suppressing a dry cough, the powdered form will be the best way to go. Mix about two teaspoons of the licorice root powder with a small amount of honey. The licorice root will sooth the inflamed throat and the honey will once again coat the throat with a layer of lubrication. Do this three times a day for as long as the cough lasts.

"The normal experience of the body and its aging is a conditioned response--a habit of thinking and behavior. By changing your habits of thinking and behavior, you can change the experience of your body and its aging." Deepak Chopra, M.D.

Everyday is a good day, if you don't believe it just try missing one.

For skin problems on your face use Cucumber, Lavender, Baby Soft, Neem Plus, or Skin Care. Pour 2 cups of boiling water over 3 to 6 drops of lavender oil. Make a steam tent with a towel and allow the steam to come up onto your face for 5 to 8 minutes. Afterwards, gently pat your face dry with a towel.

Helichrysum italicum has been successful when with skin cancer.

Another thing that may work is to dilute 10 drops of Baby Soft, or Lavender in a 2 oz. spray bottle of pure water and sprits your face several times a day. The way your body eliminates toxins is through the lungs, skin, and bowels. A healthy body will eliminate as many toxins through your skin and lungs as it will through your bowels each day. If one of your systems becomes partially clogged, the other two must take over. Many who are suffering from acne have found that when they clean out their bowels and start eating good foods their acne goes away.

Possible causes for fibromyalgia are an acid condition, mineral imbalance, vitamin E & A deficiency, and hormone imbalance. Use vitamin E and a hot compress if it is the nerves in the chest, or if it is the breast tissue use Geranium. Freedom Plus applied on location followed by Black Pepper has assisted some people. Eat foods high in the alkaline minerals of calcium, magnesium and potassium. Beneficial supplement are Ageless Plus, pH Plus, Enzymes Plus, Probiotics Plus, and Nature's Nutrients.

SOURCES

Lawless, Julia, The Encyclopedia of Essential Oils. Element, Inc., 1992

Worwood, Valerie Ann, The Complete Book of Essential Oils and Aromatherapy. New World Library, 1991

Valnet, M.D., Jean, The Practice of Aromatherapy. Destiny Books, 1982

Lavabre, Marcel, Aromatherapy Workbook. Healing Arts Presses, 1990

Burrows, Stanley, Healing for the Age of Enlightenment. Burroughs Books, 1993

Balch, M.D., James F. and Balch, C.N.C., Phyllis A., Prescription for Nutritional Healing Second Edition. Avery Publishing Group, 1997

Tolman, Don, The Water Report. 1996

LeGro, William, Reverse Aging. Glove Communications Corp, 1994

Lawren, Bill, "Calcium that 'Miracle' Mineral." Readers Digest, April, 1996

Banik, Allen E., The Choice is Clear. Acres U.S.A., 1995

Wade, Carlson, The New Enzyme-Catalyst Diet. Parker Publishing Company, Inc., 1976

Gates, Donna, The Body Ecology Diet. B.E.D. Publications, 1995

Revell, "An Introduction To Anatomy An Illustrated Guide to The Visible Man", 1977

D'Adamo, Peter J. Dr., Eat Right For Your Type. G. P. Putnam's Sons, 1996

Gramercy Books, Aunt Sally's Tried and True Home Remedies. Random House, 1993

Romain, Effie and Hawkey, Sue, Herbal Remedies, DK Publishing, Inc., 1993

Ody, Penelope, Home Herbal. Dorling Kindersley, Inc., 1995

Gary Young, Aromatherapy the Essential Beginning. Essential Press Publishing, 1996

Nittler, M.D., Alen H., A New Breed of Docter.

Pyramid House, 1972

Santillo, Humbart, B.S., M.H., Food Enzymes, The Missing Link to Radiant Health. Hohm Press, 1993

Bremness, Lesley, The Complete Book of Herbs. Viking Penguin Inc., 1988

Keller, Erich, The Complete Home Guide to Aromatherapy. H J Kramer, Inc., 1991

Penoel, M.D., Daniel and Pierre Franchomme. L'aromatherapie exactement. Limoges, France: Jollois, 1990.

Bullivant, D.Sc., ND DNM, Vaughan, The Healing Power of Herbs. Bullivan's Natural Health Products, Queensland, Australia, 1998

Lowe, Carl, Nechas, James & Editors of Prevention Magazine, Whole Body Healing. Rodale Press, Inc., 1983

Duke, James A., PhD, The Green Pharmacy. Rodale Press, 1997

Peter Schleicher, M.D., and Mohamed Saleh, M.D. Black Cumin, The Magical Egyptian Herb. Healing Arts Press a division of Inner Traditions International, 2000

Kurt Schnaubelt, PhD. Advanced Aromatherapy. Healing Art Press, 1998

Robert R. Bearfoot and Carl J. Reich, M.D. The Calcium Factor. Deanna Enterprises Publishing, 1999

Lita Lee, PhD., with Lisa Turner and Burton Goldberg. The Enzyme Cure. Future Medicine Publishing, 1998

Paavo Airola, N.D., PhD. How to Get Well. Health Plus Publishers, 1974

Schuyler W. Lininger, Jr. The Natural Pharmacy. Prima Publishing, 1998

Joni Keim Loughran and Ruah Bull. Aromatherapy and Subtle Energy Techniques.

About the Author

Bevonne has studied and worked with herbs for over 45 years. She used herbs extensively as she raised her seven children. Bevonne found that using herb teas as the base for the baby formula for her triplets really made a difference. If they had colic, diarrhea, or a runny nose, the herbs took care of the problem.

From 1974 to 1976 Bevonne owned and managed Suttler's Loft, a health food store in Franklin, Tennessee. Over the years her knowledge grew through numerous classes, hands-on experience and self- education. In 1992 while attending a Preparedness Expo in Salt Lake City, Utah she was introduced and fell in love with the essential oils.

In the summer of 1993, Bevonne and her husband, Rex, volunteered on an herb farm in St. Maries, Idaho. This gave them first hand experience in growing and distilling the plants. Aside from over 22 years of personal use and experience with the oils, Bevonne has attended over 400 hours of workshops, seminars, and conventions. Some of her instructors include: Philippe Mailhebiau, owner of Phytosun' Aromas, one of the few laboratories certified by the French government; Jean Claude Lapraz, MD. a sought after lecturer on essential oils; Daniel Penoel, MD, internationally acclaimed expert on oils and their clinical application; D. Gary Young, owner of several essential oil farms, lecturer and author; Valerie Worwood, author of several essential oil books; and John Lee, M.D. who has pioneered the research on progesterone cream and its benefits.

From 1993 to 1995 she and her husband served a church mission in the Philippines. Due to the lack of available medical services, Bevonne gained practical experience with the oils as she administered them to the people among whom she lived. She personally saw how the oils assisted in childbirth, dehydration, skin problems, parasites, and healing broken bones.

In August of 1996 she published Bevonne's Notebook, a compilation of her notes and personal experiences. In October of 1996, Bevonne and Rex attended Dr. Young's two-week course on essential oils in Izmir, Turkey sponsored by The Ege University.

From March 1999 to August 2000 Bevonne & Rex served another mission in Ghana, West Africa. Here again the oils were very useful not only in helping them but also the people in the areas where they lived. In Ghana they were introduced to the healing properties of Neem. The benefits of this plant have been used for centuries in Africa. You will find Neem in Neem Plus and Freedom Plus, two of Bevonne's favorites.

In April 2001 she updated and revised her notebook to Your Guide to Essential Oils, Minerals and Nutrition. Bevonne feels the therapeutic essential oils and minerals are wonderful companions for building health. In May 2003 Rex passed away. Bevonne is continuing to carry on the work they started together.

In 2004 the US Government passed the CAFTA law making essential oils an over-the-counter drug. The law states that unless you are a Native American Medicine Man or Woman or a Medical Doctor it is against the CAFTA law to use the term essential oils when speaking about the healing properties of the plants. Bevonne was adopted as a Native American Medicine Woman in July of 2003 and started using the word "copal" meaning herb and "liquid copal" which stands for essential oils. This way she can share the healing benefits of the plants as she speaks about the sacred traditional ways of using the copals. As a Medicine Woman she can continue teaching about the liquid copals.

In September 2006 through July 2007, her project was to prepare five Training Kits that would contain a Workbook, CD or DVD. It has been one of Bevonne's dreams (even though it was extremely hard to get her to appear on camera) to produce material to benefit more people in learning about the traditional healing properties and uses of the essential oils. She expresses the hope that these

Kits will make it easier for those wishing to learn about the many benefits of the essential oils. With the new oils and name changes in 2014 some of these Kits and Workbooks are being updated.

- The Basic Training Kits includes a workbook and CD that covers the 20 essential oils in the Basic I and Basic II Kits. It explains important information about the use of essential oils for those just getting started. It discusses way the oils may be used and some of the applications for using them.

- The Emotional Training Kit contains a workbook and DVD. It discusses the ways essential oils are used in dealing with emotions. We learn that the sense of smell is 10,000 to 100,000 times more beneficial for releasing emotions than all our other senses put together. On the DVD are demonstrations on how to use the oils to release emotions. The training kit also teaches about the benefits of the ten oils that are in the Emotional Kit.

- The Rejuvenation Training Kit contains a workbook and DVD covers ten more of the essential oils and goes into some of the applications for using them. The simplified version of Vita Flex is taught in this training. The Vita Flex application assists in reducing stress and tension while rejuvenating and relaxing the body. This is a technique many massage therapists use and now you can use it to benefit your family. The training DVD also shows an application that has been known to be beneficial for hearing problems.

- The Prosperity Training Kit contains a DVD and Workbook that explains how essential oils have a frequency that draws to us what we focus on. We learn how we need to prepare ourselves for prosperity by eliminating what has been holding us back.

Our fears have the tendency to sabotage our progress. It also explains how certain letters in your handwriting actually can hinder the achievement of your goals. It shows you how to change those letters to benefit your life. The Workbook explains how people who have become prosperous have had goals to direct them. It gives assignments that will assist you in your progress. This training kit also discusses the ten essential oils found in the Prosperity Kit, their benefits and the application.

- The Handwriting Training Kit teaches the correct way of writing each letter of the alphabet. The most important letter to write correctly is the "I". The way it is written indicates how you get along with people. When the "I" is written backwards it brings an attitude of despair, arguing, frustration, and imbalance into the life of the writer. The book and DVD discusses what the benefits of forming your letters correctly could be for the writer. The Workbook is entitled *Change you Handwriting, Change your Life*.

In 2007 Bevonne updated her Workbook again and renamed it *The Healing Power of Liquid Copals* to become compliant with the US Government regulations and incorporate the Native American sacred traditional term "liquid copal." Since then new liquid copals and information has been added to the Workbook from time to time.

In 2009 Bevonne was adopted into the Oklevueha Native American Band in Ava, Missouri. She is now working with that Band.

In September of 2012 Bevonne married David Crookston and together they are teaching about the healing power of essential oils. Bevonne hopes this workbook will help you learn about the essential oils and their traditional uses.

Made in the USA
Middletown, DE
29 July 2015